Basic Medical Co for Physician Practices

Cynthia Newby, CPC

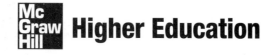

Higher Education

Boston   Burr Ridge, IL   Dubuque, IA   Madison, WI   New York   San Francisco   St. Louis
Bangkok   Bogotá   Caracas   Kuala Lumpur   Lisbon   London   Madrid   Mexico City
Milan   Montreal   New Delhi   Santiago   Seoul   Singapore   Sydney   Taipei   Toronto

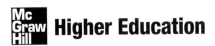

Higher Education

BASIC MEDICAL CODING FOR PHYSICIAN PRACTICES

Published by McGraw-Hill, a business unit of The McGraw-Hill Companies, Inc., 1221 Avenue of the Americas, New York, NY 10020. Copyright © 2005 by The McGraw-Hill Companies, Inc. All rights reserved. No part of this publication may be reproduced or distributed in any form or by any means, or stored in a database or retrieval system, without the prior written consent of The McGraw-Hill Companies, Inc., including, but not limited to, in any network or other electronic storage or transmission, or broadcast for distance learning.

Contains material previously published in *Medical Insurance: A Guide to Coding and Reimbursement, 2e,* Chapters 4, 5, and 6; and as *Medical Insurance Coding Workbook for Physician Practices, 2004–2005 Edition.*

Some ancillaries, including electronic and print components, may not be available to customers outside the United States.

This book is printed on recycled, acid-free paper containing 10% postconsumer waste.

1 2 3 4 5 6 7 8 9 QPD/QPD 9 8 7 6 5 4

ISBN 0–07–301832–5

Publisher: *David T. Culverwell*
Senior Sponsoring Editor: *Roxan Kinsey*
Developmental Editor: *Patricia Forrest*
Editorial Coordinator: *Connie Kuhl*
Senior Marketing Manager: *James F. Connely*
Project Manager: *Cindy Schmerbach*
Production Supervisor: *Kara Kudronowciz*
Lead Media Project Manager: *Audrey A. Reiter*
Media Technology Producer: *Janna Martin*
Designer: *Laurie B. Janssen*
Cover Designer: *Lisa Gravunder*
Cover Illustration: *Lisa Gravunder*
Supplement Producer: *Brenda A. Ernzen*
Compositor: *Lithokraft*
Typeface: *11.5/13 Minion*
Printer: *QuebecorWorld Dubuque, IA*

All brand or product names are trademarks or registered trademarks of their respective companies.

CPT five-digit codes, nomenclature, and other data are copyright 2003 American Medical Association. All Rights Reserved. No fee schedules, basic units relative values, or related listings are included in CPT. The AMA assumes no liability for the data contained herein.

CPT codes are based on CPT 2004.
ICD-9-CM codes are based on ICD-9-CM 2004.

All names, situations, and anecdotes are fictitious. They do not represent any person, event, or medical record.

www.mhhe.com

Brief Contents

Contents

PART 3 Coding Linkage and Compliance 80

To the Student

Your career as a physician practice medical coder

This class introduces you to the skills you will need for a successful career in medical coding. Medical coding specialists work in a number of health care settings, including physician practices, hospitals, government agencies, and insurance companies. Coders who work in practices review patients' medical records and assign diagnosis and procedure codes. They are knowledgeable about the coding rules and procedures for physicians' work, which are different than those for coding hospital services.

The position of medical coding specialist is growing in importance in physician practices. Accurate coding is a critical part of ensuring that claims follow the legal and ethical requirements of government programs like Medicare and other payers, as well as the federal HIPAA (Health Insurance Portability and Accountability Act) laws.

Medical office employees may gain required health care work experience and then attain coding positions through coding education from seminars or college classes. Certification as a professional coder offers an excellent route to success as a medical coder in the medical practice setting. Some employers require certification for employment; others state that certification must be earned after a certain amount of time in the position, such as six months. Coding classes followed by examinations are used to obtain certification. These physician-office coding certifications are available:

- The American Health Information Management Association (AHIMA) offers the Certified Coding Associate (CCA) credential and the Certified Coding Specialist—Physician-based (CCS-P) credential. The CCA is an entry-level title; completion of either a training program or six months' job experience is recommended. The CCS-P requires at least three years of coding experience.

- The American Academy of Professional Coders (AAPC) offers the Certified Professional Coder (CPC) credential, also requiring coursework and on-the-job experience, and an associate level, the CPC-A.

If you have a coding credential as well as coding experience, you may have the opportunity to advance to coding management and coding compliance auditor positions. Becoming expert in a specialty such as surgical coding also offers advancement opportunities.

How can I succeed in this class, a first step toward my goals?

If you're reading this, you're on the right track.

"You are the same today that you are going to be five years from now except for two things: the people with whom you associate and the books you read."

Charles Jones

Right now, you're probably leafing through this book feeling just a little overwhelmed. You're trying to juggle several other classes (which probably are equally as intimidating), possibly a job, and on top of it all, a life.

It's true—you are what you put into your studies. You have a lot of time and money invested in your education. Don't blow it now by only putting in half of the effort this class requires. Succeeding in this class (and life) requires:

- **A commitment—of time and perseverance**
- **Knowing and motivating yourself**
- **Getting organized**
- **Managing your time**

This special introduction has been designed specifically to help you focus. It's here to help you learn how to manage your time and your studies to succeed. It will help you learn how to be effective in these areas, as well as offer guidance in:

- **Getting the most out of your lecture**
- **Thinking through—and applying—the material**
- **Getting the most out of your textbook**
- **Finding extra help when you need it**

A commitment—of time and perseverance

Learning—and mastering—takes time. And patience. Nothing worthwhile comes easily. Be committed to your studies and you will reap the benefits in the long run.

Consider this: your coding courses are building the foundation for your future—a future in your chosen profession. Sloppy and hurried craftsmanship now will only lead to ruins later.

STUDY TIP *A good rule of thumb is to allow 2 hours of study time for every hour you spend in lecture.*

Knowing and motivating yourself

What type of a learner are you? When are you most productive? Know yourself and your limits and work within them. Know how to motivate yourself to give your all to your studies and achieve your goals. Quite bluntly, you are the one that benefits most from your success. If you lack self-motivation and drive, you are the first person that suffers.

Knowing yourself—There are many types of learners, and no right or wrong way of learning. Which category do you fall into?

- Visual learner—You respond best to "seeing" processes and information. Particularly focus on the text's examples and hints.
- Auditory learner—You work best by listening to—and possibly tape recording–the lecture and by talking information through with a study partner.
- Tactile / Kinesthetic Learner—You learn best by being "hands on." You'll benefit by applying what you've learned during lab time. Think of how to apply your critical thinking skills. Perhaps a text website will also help you.

Identify your own personal preferences for learning and seek out the resources that will best help you with your studies. Also, learn by recognizing your weaknesses and try to compensate/work to improve them.

Getting organized

It's simple, yet it's fundamental. It seems the more organized you are, the easier things come. Take the time before your course begins to look around and analyze your life and your study habits. Get organized now and you'll find you have a little more time—and a lot less stress.

Find a calendar system that works for you. The best kind is one that you can take with you everywhere. To be truly organized, you should integrate all aspects of your life into this one calendar—school, work, leisure. Some people also find it helpful to have an additional monthly calendar posted by their desk for "at a glance" dates and to have a visual of what's to come. If you do this, be sure you are consistently synchronizing both calendars as not to miss anything. More tips for organizing your calendar can be found in the time management discussion below.

By the same token, keep everything for your course or courses in one place—and at your fingertips. A three-ring binder works well because it allows you to add or organize handouts and notes from class in any order you prefer. Incorporating your own custom tabs helps you flip to exactly what you need at a moments notice.

Find your space. Find a place that helps you be organized and focused. If it's your desk in your dorm room or in your home, keep it clean. Clutter adds confusion, stress, and wastes time. Or perhaps your "space" is at the library. If that's the case, keep a backpack or bag that's fully stocked with what you might need—your text, binder or notes, pens, highlighters, Post-its, phone numbers of study partners (hint: a good place to keep phone numbers is in your "one place for everything calendar").

A HELPFUL HINT—*add extra "padding" into your deadlines to yourself. If you have a report due on Friday, set a goal for yourself to have it done on Wednesday. Then, take time on Thursday to look over your project again, with a fresh eye. Make any corrections or enhancements and have it ready to turn in on Friday.*

Managing your time

Managing your time is the single most important thing you can do to help yourself. And, it's probably one of the most difficult tasks to successfully master.

You are taking this course because you want to succeed in life. You are preparing for a career. You are expected to work much harder and to learn much more than you ever have before. To be successful you need to invest in your education with a commitment of time.

How time slips away
People tend to let an enormous amount of time slip away from them, mainly in three ways:

- **procrastination**, putting off chores simply because we don't feel in the mood to do them right away
- **distraction**, getting sidetracked by the endless variety of other things that seem easier or more fun to do, often not realizing how much time they eat up
- **underestimating the value of small bits of time**, thinking it's not worth doing any work because we have something else to do or somewhere else to be in 20 minutes or so.

We all lead busy lives. But we all make choices as to how we spend our time. Choose wisely and make the most of every minute you have by implementing these tips.

Know yourself and when you'll be able to study most efficiently.
When are you most productive? Are you a late nighter? Or an early bird? Plan to study when you are most alert and can have uninterrupted segments. This could include a quick 5-minute review before class or a one-hour problem solving study session with a friend.

Create a set study time for yourself daily.
Having a set schedule for yourself helps you commit to studying, and helps you plan instead of cram. Find—and use—a planner that is small enough that you can take with you—everywhere. This can be a $2.50 paper calendar or a more expensive electronic version. They all work on the same premise—*organize all of your activities in one place.*

Make sure you log your projects and homework deadlines in your personal calendar.

Less is more. Schedule study time using shorter, focused blocks with small breaks. Doing this offers two benefits:

1. You will be less fatigued and gain more from your effort, and
2. Studying will seem less overwhelming and you will be less likely to procrastinate.

Plan time for leisure, friends, exercise, and sleep.
Studying should be your main focus, but you need to balance your time—and your life.

Try to complete tasks ahead of schedule. This will give you a chance to carefully review your work before you hand it in (instead of at 1 a.m. when you are half awake). You'll feel less stressed in the end.

Prioritize!

In your calendar or planner, highlight or number key projects; do them first, and then cross them off when you've completed them. Give yourself a pat on the back for getting them done! Review your calendar and reprioritize daily.

Try to resist distractions by setting and sticking to a designated study time (remember your commitment and perseverance!) Distractions may include friends and surfing the Internet…

Multitask when possible

You may find a lot of extra time you didn't think you had. Review material or organize your term paper in your head while walking to class, doing laundry, or during "mental down time." (Note—mental down time does NOT mean in the middle of lecture.)

Getting the most out of lectures

Believe it or not, instructors want you to succeed. They put a lot of effort into helping you learn and preparing their lectures. Attending class is one of the simplest, most valuable things you can do to help yourself. But it doesn't end there . . . getting the most out of your lectures means being organized. Here's how:

Prepare before you go to class

Really! You'll be amazed at how much more comprehensible the material will be when you preview the chapter before you go to class. Don't feel overwhelmed by this already. One tip that may help you—plan to arrive to class 5-15 minutes before lecture. Bring your text with you and skim the chapter before lecture begins. This will at the very least give you an overview of what may be discussed.

Be a good listener

Most people think they are good listeners, but few really are. Are you?

Obvious, but important points to remember:

- You can't listen if you are talking.

- You aren't listening if you are daydreaming.

- Listening and comprehending are two different things. If you don't understand something your instructor is saying, ask a question or jot a note and visit the instructor after hours. Don't feel dumb or intimidated; you probably aren't the only person who "doesn't get it."

Take good notes

- Use a standard size notebook, and better yet, a three-ring binder with loose leaf notepaper. The binder will allow you to organize and integrate your notes and handouts, integrate easy-to-reference tabs, etc.

- Use a standard black or blue ink pen to take your initial notes. You can annotate later using a pencil, which can be erased if need be.
- Start a new page with each lecture or note taking session (yes—you can and should also take notes from your textbook).
- Label each page with the date and a heading for each day.
- Focus on main points and try to use an outline format to take notes to capture key ideas and organize sub-points.
- Review and edit your notes shortly after class—at least within 24 hours—to make sure they make sense and that you've recorded core thoughts. You may also want to compare your notes with a study partner later to make sure neither of you have missed anything.

<u>Get a study partner</u>

Having a study partner has so many benefits. First, he/she can help you keep your commitment to this class. By having set study dates, you can combine study and social time, and maybe even make it fun! In addition, you now have two sets of eyes and ears and two minds to help digest the information from lecture and from the text. Talk through concepts, compare notes, and quiz each other.

An obvious note: Don't take advantage of your study partner by skipping class or skipping study dates. You obviously won't have a study partner—or a friend—much longer if it's not a mutually beneficial arrangement!

HELPFUL HINT: *Take your text to lecture, and keep it open to the topics being discussed. You can take brief notes in your textbook margin or reference textbook pages in your notebook to help you study later.*

Getting the most out of your textbook

McGraw-Hill and the author of this book, Cynthia, have invested our time, research, and talents to help you succeed as well. Our goal is to make learning—for you—easier.

Here's how.

The text has three instructional parts. Each opens with

- Objectives, so you understand the key points you should master.
- Key Terms, so you begin to build your medical coding vocabulary.
- Why This Part Is Important to You, to explain the purpose of the material you are about to learn.

The text also has a part with coding worksheets. After you study the related text material, try answering the questions on the worksheet you have been asked to complete. If any of your answers are incorrect, study that material again to see what you missed the first time. Coding is about learning and practice!

The text ends with Coding Quizzes. These items help you test your knowledge of the concepts and applications you have learned in the related part. They also give you experience with the format of the national associations' coding certification exams.

To the Instructor

Basic Medical Coding is designed for entry-level students who have a background in medical terminology and anatomy/physiology. The text/workbook combines material previously published as Chapters 4, 5, and 6 of McGraw-Hill's *Medical Insurance: A Guide to Coding and Reimbursement, 2e,* combined with the *Medical Insurance Coding Workbook for Physician Practices.*

Using *Basic Medical Coding,* students will learn the structure and conventions of ICD-9-CM and CPT, the correct process for selecting codes, and the types of coding errors to be avoided.

The Instructor's Manual contains the answers to the worksheet exercises and quizzes. It also contains a CD-ROM with two tools to enhance the instructional process, the Instructor's Presentation Software—a PowerPoint presentation of Parts 1, 2, and 3 of the program—and assessment software, an ExamView Pro Testbank that allows instructors to create, edit, and print customized tests for each part.

The technical reviewers acknowledged below offered invaluable assistance in reviewing the manuscript, exercises, and answers for accuracy. The reviewers and I hope that we have been correct in our work. Any errors, however, are the author's responsbililty. You are encouraged to report these to McGraw-Hill Higher Education, so that corrections can be made.

Technical Reviewers

Daphne Balacos, CPC

Ms. Balacos has a Bachelor of Science degree from the University of New Haven and has been in the health care field since 1984. She is currently a consultant specializing in CPT, ICD, and HCPCS education. A Certified Professional Coder (CPC) and cofounder of the Connecticut Chapter of the American Academy of Professional Coders (AAPC), Ms. Balacos has been a presenter at national coding conferences and is an approved instructor of the AAPCs Professional Medical Coding Curriculum (PMCC).

Sheryl L. Fritz, RHIT, CCS-P

Ms. Fritz has worked in the health care field for over twenty years. She is currently the compliance specialist for the Office of Professional Services of Hartford Hospital in Hartford, CT. In this position, she is responsible for all coding and documentation compliance activities for thirty hospital-based specialty physician group practices as well as the hospital's ambulatory medicine practice. A Certified Coding Specialist-Physician-based (CCS-P) and Registered Health Information Technician, Ms. Fritz is active in the American Health Information Management Association (AHIMA) and the Connecticut Health Information Management Association, for which she serves on the board of directors.

Mary E. Halstead, LPL, CPC

Ms. Halstead is a Licensed Practical Nurse (LPN). She has worked as a staff nurse and staff coordinator for health care facilities and as a utilization review nurse and health service referral nurse for major medical insurance companies. Currently, she is the data quality reviewer of Coventry Health Care in West Des Moines, lA, where she reviews claims for coding accuracy, assesses documentation for support of claims, determines the coverage of benefits, and meets with providers to resolve issues concerning claims or coding. She is a Certified Professional Coder (CPC) by the American Academy of Professional Coders (AAPC) and is an active member of the Central Iowa Chapter of the AAPC.

Amy L. Wood, CPC

Amy Wood has held a variety of positions in the health information field. She has supervised the billing and coding functions at a multi-physician specialty practice. For Yale New Haven Hospital, New Haven, CT, she was a coding compliance analyst, serving as the APC specialist and acting as a liaison for resolving billing and coding issues for this 900+ bed hospital.

Ms. Wood is currently Business Office Site Coordinator in the Systems Business Office for Yale New Haven Hospital. In this role, she is directing an initiative that is aimed at redefining coders' functions. The goal of this change is to improve charge capture by placing coders in the hospital's departments, where they will assign both codes based on documentation in the medical record as well as charges through the charge description master.

A Certified Professional Coder (CPC), Ms. Wood is a member of the Connecticut Chapter of the American Academy of Professional Coders (AAPC).

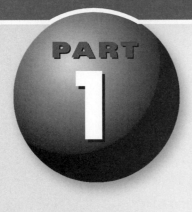

PART 1

Coding Diagnoses

Objectives

After studying this part, you will be able to:

1. Discuss the purpose of the ICD-9-CM.
2. Describe the structure and content of the Alphabetic Index and the Tabular List.
3. Interpret the conventions that are followed in the Alphabetic Index and the Tabular List.
4. Identify the purpose and correct use of V codes and E codes.
5. List the three steps in the diagnostic coding process.
6. Describe and provide examples of three key coding guidelines.
7. Analyze diagnostic statements, apply appropriate coding guidelines, and assign correct ICD-9-CM codes.

Key Terms

acute
adverse effect
Alphabetic Index
category
chronic
coexisting condition
combination code
convention
diagnostic statement
E code

eponym
etiology
ICD-9-CM
late effect
main term
manifestation
NEC (not elsewhere classified)
NOS (not otherwise specified)

primary diagnosis
subcategory
subclassification
subterm
supplementary term
Tabular List
unspecified
V code

Why This Part Is Important to You

For more than a hundred years, scientists and researchers have gathered information from hospital records about patients' illnesses and causes of death. Because people have many different symptoms and conditions, a standard system of diagnosis codes has been developed for recording them. A coding system provides an accurate way to collect statistics to keep people healthy and to plan for needed resources, as well as to record morbidity (disease) and mortality (death) data.

In physicians' practices, diagnosis codes are used to report patients' conditions on health care claims. The physicians, medical coders, insurance/billing specialists, or medical assistants may be responsible for assigning the codes. Expertise in diagnostic coding requires knowledge of medical terminology, anatomy and physiology, and pathophysiology, as well as experience in correctly applying the rules of the coding system.

This part of *Basic Medical Coding* gives you a fundamental understanding of current diagnostic coding principles and guidelines. You also have an opportunity to reinforce this understanding by practicing your coding skills as you complete the Coding Worksheets and take the ICD Coding Quiz. The goal is to enable you to work effectively with encounter forms and health care claims.

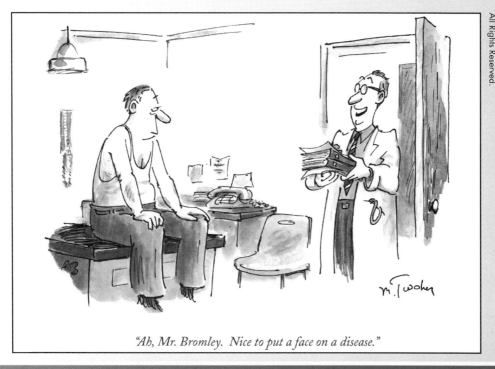

"Ah, Mr. Bromley. Nice to put a face on a disease."

The diagnosis codes used in the United States are based on the *International Classification of Diseases* (ICD). The ICD lists diseases and their three-digit codes according to a system created by the World Health Organization of the United Nations. It has been revised a number of times since the coding system was first developed.

History

A U.S. version of the ninth edition of the ICD (ICD-9) was published in 1979. A committee of physicians from various organizations and specialties prepared this version, which is called the ICD-9's *Clinical Modification*, or ICD-9-CM. Codes in the ICD-9-CM describe conditions and illnesses more precisely than does the World Health Organization's ICD-9 because the codes are intended to provide a more complete picture of patients' conditions. The Medicare Catastrophic Coverage Act of 1988 mandated the change from written diagnoses to ICD-9-CM diagnosis codes for Medicare claims. After the Medicare ruling, private payers also began to require physicians to report diagnoses with ICD-9-CM codes. The use of these diagnosis codes in the health care industry is now standard.

ICD-9-CM diagnosis codes are made up of three, four, or five digits, and a description. The system uses three-digit categories for diseases, injuries, and symptoms. Many of these categories are subcategorized into four-digit codes. Some codes are further subdivided into five-digit codes. For example:

> Category 415: Acute pulmonary heart disease (three digits)
>> Subcategory 415.1: Pulmonary embolism and infarction (four digits)
>>> Subclassification: 415.11: Iatrogenic pulmonary embolism and infarction (five digits)

The purpose of the fourth-level and fifth-level diagnosis codes is to record the most specific diagnosis documented in the patient medical record. When included in the ICD-9-CM, fourth and fifth digits are not optional; they must be used. For example, current Centers for Medicare and Medicaid Services (CMS) rules state that a Medicare claim will be rejected when the most specific code available is not used.

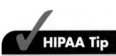

HIPAA Tip

Mandated Use of ICD-9-CM

- ICD-9-CM is the mandated code set for physician services under HIPAA's Electronic Health Care Transactions and Code Sets.
- ICD-9-CM diagnosis codes must be included on all Medicare electronic and paper health care claims for physicians' services.

Keeping Codes Up to Date

When the new codes are received, office forms and billing software must be readied. HIPAA rules require health care claims to report the codes that were current on the date of service—not the date the claim is prepared.

Updates

The National Center for Health Statistics and the CMS release updates for the ICD-9-CM on April 1 and October 1 of every year. New codes must be used as of the release date. The U.S. Government Printing Office (GPO) publishes the official ICD-9-CM on the Internet and in CD-ROM format. Various commercial publishers present the updated codes in annual coding books that are also available soon after the addenda are released. Practices must ensure that the current reference is available and that the current codes are in use.

NEW REVISION: THE ICD-10-CM

A new *Clinical Modification* (ICD-10-CM) is being reviewed by health care professionals. It is expected to be adopted as the mandatory diagnosis code set to replace ICD-9-CM before 2010. The major changes include the following:

- ICD-10-CM contains over 2,000 categories of diseases, many more than the ICD-9-CM. This creates more codes to permit more specific reporting of diseases and newly recognized conditions.
- Codes are alphanumeric, containing a letter followed by up to five numbers.
- The sixth digit is added to capture clinical details. For example, all codes that relate to pregnancy, labor, and childbirth include a digit that indicates the patient's trimester.
- Codes are added to show which side of the body is affected when a disease or condition can be involved with the right side, the left side, or bilaterally. For example, separate codes are listed for a malignant neoplasm of right upper-inner quadrant of the female breast and for a malignant neoplasm of left upper-inner quadrant of the female breast.

Although the code numbers look different, the basic systems are very much alike, and people who are familiar with the current codes will find that their training quickly applies to the new system.

Coding Point

Each year, the ICD has many new and changed codes, in part to classify the diseases that have been discovered since the previous revision. What are examples of diseases that have been diagnosed in the last two decades?

Internet Tip

Access the Web site of the National Center for Health Statistics, which has up-to-date information on ICD:

http://www.cdc.gov/nchs

Locate information on the current year's ICD-9-CM new codes. Also, research and report on the status of ICD-10-CM.

ORGANIZATION OF THE ICD-9-CM

The ICD-9-CM has three parts:

1. *Diseases and Injuries: Tabular List—Volume 1:* The **Tabular List** is made up of seventeen chapters of disease descriptions and codes, with two supplementary classifications and five appendixes.
2. *Diseases and Injuries: Alphabetic Index—Volume 2:* The **Alphabetic Index** provides (a) an index of the disease descriptions in the Tabular List, (b) an index in table format of drugs and chemicals that cause poisoning, and (c) an index of external causes of injury, such as accidents.

3. *Procedures: Tabular List and Alphabetic Index—Volume 3:* This volume covers procedures performed by physicians and other practitioners, chiefly in hospitals.

Volumes 1 and 2 are used for physician practice (outpatient) diagnostic coding.

Although the Tabular List and the Alphabetic Index are labeled Volume 1 and Volume 2, they are related like the parts of a book. The chapters in the Tabular List are followed by an index. First, the Alphabetic Index is used to find a code for a patient's condition or symptom. The index entry provides a pointer to the correct code number in the Tabular List. Then, that code is located in the Tabular List so that its correct use can be checked. This two-step process must be followed in order to code correctly. This chapter follows this order of use, with the Alphabetic Index discussed first, followed by the Tabular List. (Some publishers' versions of the ICD-9-CM place the Alphabetic Index before the Tabular List for the same reason.)

THE ALPHABETIC INDEX

The Alphabetic Index contains all the medical terms in the Tabular List classifications. For some conditions, it also lists common terms that are not found in the Tabular List. The index is organized by the condition, not by the body part (anatomical site) in which it occurs. For example, the term *wrist fracture* is located by looking under *fracture* (the condition) and then, below it, *wrist* (the location), rather than under *wrist* to find *fracture.*

The medical term describing the condition for which a patient is receiving care is located in the physician's **diagnostic statement.** For each encounter, the diagnostic statement includes the main reason for the patient encounter. It may also provide descriptions of additional conditions or symptoms that have been treated or that are related to the patient's current illness.

Main Terms, Subterms, and Supplementary Terms

The assignment of the correct code begins with looking up the medical term that describes the patient's condition. Figure 1.1 shows the format of the Alphabetic Index. Each **main term** is printed in boldface type and is followed by its code number. For example, if the diagnostic statement is "the patient presents with blindness," the main term *blindness* is located in the Alphabetic Index (see Figure 1.1).

Below the main term, any **subterms** with their codes appear. Subterms are essential in the selection of correct codes. They may show the **etiology** of the disease—its cause or origin—or describe a particular type or body site for the main term. For example, the main term *blindness* in Figure 1.1 includes five subterms, each indicating a different etiology or type—such as color blindness—for that condition.

Any **supplementary terms** for main terms or subterms are shown in parentheses on the same line. Supplementary terms are not essential to the selection of the correct code, and are often referred to as nonessential

Blepharitis (eyelid) 373.00
  angularis 373.01
  ciliaris 373.00
   with ulcer 373.01
  marginal 373.00
   with ulcer 373.01
  scrofulous (*see also* Tuberculosis) 017.3
   [373.00]
  squamous 373.02
  ulcerative 373.01
Blepharochalasis 374.34
  congenital 743.62
Blepharoclonus 333.81
Blepharoconjunctivitis (*see also* Conjunctivitis)
  372.20
  angular 372.21
  contact 372.22
Blepharophimosis (eyelid) 374.46
  congenital 743.62
Blepharoplegia 374.89
Blepharoptosis 374.30
  congenital 743.61
Blepharopyorrhea 098.49
Blepharospasm 333.81

Blessig's cyst 362.62
Blighted ovum 631
Blind
  bronchus (congenital) 748.3
  eye—*see also* Blindness
   hypertensive 360.42
   hypotensive 360.41
  loop syndrome (postoperative) 579.2
  sac, fallopian tube (congenital) 752.19
  spot, enlarged 368.42
  tract or tube (congenital) NEC—*see* Atresia
Blindness (acquired) (congenital) (Both eyes)
  369.00
  blast 921.3
   with nerve injury—*see* Injury, nerve, optic
  Brightís — *see* Uremia
  color (congenital) 368.59
   acquired 368.55
   blue 368.53
   green 368.52
   red 368.51
   total 368.54
  concussion 950.9
  cortical 377.75

FIGURE 1.1 Example of Alphabetic Index Entries

modifiers. They help point to the correct term, but they do not have to appear in the physician's diagnostic statement for the coder to correctly select the code. In Figure 1.1, for example, any of the supplementary terms *acquired, congenital,* and *both eyes* may modify the main term in the diagnostic statement, such as "the patient presents with blindness acquired in childhood," or none of these terms may appear.

Turnover Lines

If the main term or subterm is too long to fit on one line, as is often the case when many supplementary terms appear, turnover (or carryover) lines are used. Turnover lines are always indented farther to the right than are subterms. It is important to read carefully to distinguish a turnover line from a subterm line. For example, under the main term *blindness* (Figure 1.1) in the Alphabetic Index, a long list of supplementary terms appears before the first subterm. Without close attention, it is possible to confuse a turnover entry with a subterm.

Cross-References

Some entries use cross-references. If the cross-reference *see* appears after a main term, the coder *must* look up the term that follows the word *see* in the index. The *see* reference means that the main term where the coder first looked is not correct; another category must be used. In Figure 1.1, for example, to code the last subterm under *blind*, the term *atresia* must be found.

See also, another type of cross-reference, points the coder to additional, related index entries. *See also category* indicates that the coder should review the additional categories that are mentioned. For example, in the following entry, the entries between 633.0 and 633.9 should be checked, as well as 639.0:

Sepsis with ectopic pregnancy (*see also categories* 633.0–633.9) 639.0

Notes

At times, notes are shown below terms. These boxed, italicized instructions are important because they provide information on selecting the correct code. For example, this note appears in the listings for inguinal hernias (category 550):

> *Note—Use the following fifth-digit subclassification with category 550:*
>
> *0   unilateral or unspecified (not specified as recurrent)*
>
> *1   unilateral or unspecified, recurrent*
>
> *2   bilateral (not specified as recurrent)*
>
> *3   bilateral, recurrent*

This note also illustrates another **convention** that is followed in the index: Numbered items are listed in numerical order from lowest to highest. Conventions are typographic techniques or standard practices that provide visual guidelines for understanding printed material. For example, listing numbered items in numerical order is followed whether the items are pure numbers (1, 2, 3) or words (first, second, third).

The Abbreviation NEC

Not elsewhere classified, or NEC, appears with a term when there is no code that is specific for the condition. Use of this abbreviation indicates that regardless of the information available, no code matches the particular situation. For example:

Hemorrhage, brain, traumatic NEC 853.0

Multiple Codes and Connecting Words

Some conditions may require two codes, one for the etiology and a second for the **manifestation**, the disease's typical signs or symptoms. This requirement is indicated when two codes, the second in brackets and italics, appear after a term:

Phlebitis
    gouty 274.89 *[451.9]*

This entry indicates that the diagnostic statement "gouty phlebitis" requires two codes, one for the etiology (gout) and one for the manifestation (phlebitis). The use of italics for codes means that they cannot be used as primary codes; they are listed after the codes for the etiology.

The use of connecting words, such as *due to*, *during*, *following*, and *with*, may also indicate the need for two codes, or for a single code that covers both conditions. For example, the main term below is followed by a *due to* subterm:

Cowpox (abortive) 051.0
  due to vaccination 999.0

When the Alphabetic Index indicates the possible need for two codes, the Tabular List entry is used to determine whether they are needed. In some cases, a **combination code** describing both the etiology and the manifestation is available instead of two codes. For example:

Closed skull fracture with subdural hemorrhage and concussion 803.29

Common Terms

Many terms appear more than once in the Alphabetic Index. Often, the term in common use is listed, as well as the accepted medical terminology. For example, there is an entry for *flu*, with a cross-reference to *influenza*.

Eponyms

An **eponym** is a condition (or a procedure) named for a person. Some eponyms are named for the physicians who discovered or invented them; others are named for patients. An eponym is usually listed both under that name and under the main term *disease* or *syndrome*. For example, Hodgkin's disease appears as a subterm under *disease* and as a key term.

THE TABULAR LIST

The Tabular List received its name from the language of statistics; the word *tabulate* means to count, record, or list systematically. The diseases and injuries in the Tabular List are organized into chapters according to etiology or body system. Supplementary codes and appendixes cover other special situations. The organization of the Tabular List and the ranges of codes each part covers are shown in Table 1.1 on page 10.

Categories, Subcategories, and Subclassifications

Each Tabular List chapter is divided into sections with titles that indicate the types of related disease or conditions they cover. For example, Chapter 9 has seven sections, one of which is

Hernia of Abdominal Cavity (550–553)

Within each section, there are three levels of codes:

1. A **category** is a three-digit code that covers a single disease or related condition. (See Appendix E of the Tabular List for the complete listing of categories.) For example, the category 551 in Figure 1.2 (on page 11) covers "other hernia of abdominal cavity, with gangrene."

TABLE 1.1 Tabular List Organization

Classification of Diseases and Injuries

Chapter		Categories
1	Infectious and Parasitic Diseases	001–139
2	Neoplasms	140–239
3	Endocrine, Nutritional, and Metabolic Diseases, and Immunity Disorders	240–279
4	Diseases of the Blood and Blood-Forming Organs	280–289
5	Mental Disorders	290–319
6	Diseases of the Central Nervous System and Sense Organs	320–389
7	Diseases of the Circulatory System	390–459
8	Diseases of the Respiratory System	460–519
9	Diseases of the Digestive System	520–579
10	Diseases of the Genitourinary System	580–629
11	Complications of Pregnancy, Childbirth, and the Puerperium	630–677
12	Diseases of the Skin and Subcutaneous Tissue	680–709
13	Diseases of the Musculoskeletal System and Connective Tissue	710–739
14	Congenital Anomalies	740–759
15	Certain Conditions Originating in the Perinatal Period	760–779
16	Symptoms, Signs, and Ill-Defined Conditions	780–799
17	Injury and Poisoning	800–999

Supplementary Classifications

V Codes	Supplementary Classification of Factors Influencing Health Status and Contact with Health Services	V01–V83
E Codes	Supplementary Classification of External Causes of Injury and Poisoning	E800–E999

Appendixes

Appendix A	Morphology of Neoplasms
Appendix B	Glossary of Mental Disorders
Appendix C	Classification of Drugs by American Hospital Formulary Services List Number and Their ICD-9-CM Equivalents
Appendix D	Classification of Industrial Accidents According to Agency
Appendix E	List of Three-Digit Categories

2. A **subcategory** is a four-digit subdivision of a category. It provides a further breakdown of the disease to show its etiology, site, or manifestation. For example, the 551 category has six subcategories:

551.0   Femoral hernia with gangrene

551.1   Umbilical hernia with gangrene

551.2   Ventral hernia with gangrene

551.3   Diaphragmatic hernia with gangrene

551.8   Hernia of other specified sites, with gangrene

551.9   Hernia of unspecified site, with gangrene

551 **Other hernia of abdominal cavity, with gangrene**
Includes: that with gangrene (and obstruction)

⑤ • **551.0** **Femoral hernia with gangrene**
551.00 **Unilateral or unspecified (not specified as recurrent)**
Femoral hernia NOS with gangrene
551.01 **Unilateral or unspecified, recurrent**
551.02 **Bilateral (not specified as recurrent)**
551.03 **Bilateral, recurrent**
551.1 **Umbilical hernia with gangrene**
Parumbilical hernia specified as gangrenous

⑤ • **551.2** **Ventral hernia with gangrene**
551.20 **Ventral, unspecified, with gangrene**
551.21 **Incisional, with gangrene**
Hernia:
postoperative } specified as gangrenous
Recurrent, ventral
551.29 **Other**
Epigastric hernia specified as gangrenous
551.3 **Diaphragmatic hernia with gangrene**
Hernia:
hiatal (esophageal) (sliding)
Paraesophageal } specified as gangrenous
Thoracic stomach
Excludes: *congenital diaphragmatic hernia (756.6)*

551.8 **Hernia of other specified sites, with gangrene**
Any condition classifiable to 553.8 if specified as gangrenous
551.9 **Hernia of unspecified site, with gangrene**
Any condition classifiable to 553.9 if specified as gangrenous

FIGURE 1.2 Example of Tabular List Entries

3. A **subclassification** is a five-digit subdivision of a subcategory. For example, the following fifth digits are to be used with code 551.0:

551.00 Unilateral or unspecified (not specified as recurrent)

551.01 Unilateral or unspecified, recurrent

551.02 Bilateral (not specified as recurrent)

551.03 Bilateral, recurrent

Symbols, Notes, Punctuation Marks, and Abbreviations

Coding correctly requires understanding the conventions—the symbols, instructional notes, and punctuation marks—that appear in the Tabular List.

Symbol for Fifth-Digit Requirement

Depending on the publisher of the ICD-9-CM, a section mark (§) or other symbol (such as ⑤ or ✓) appears next to a chapter, a category, or a subcategory that requires a fifth digit to be assigned. (See, for example, the ⑤ that appears next to subcategories 551.0 and 551.2 in Figure 1.2.) These are important reminders to assign the appropriate five-digit subclassification. If the fifth-digit requirement extends beyond the page where this symbol first appears, the symbol is repeated on all other pages where it applies, so that it is easy to notice.

Includes and Excludes Notes

Notes headed by the word *includes* refine the content of the category or section appearing above them. For example, after the three-digit category 461, acute sinusitis, the *include* note states that the category includes abscess, empyema, infection, inflammation, and suppuration.

Notes headed by the word *excludes* (which is boxed and italicized) indicate conditions that are not classifiable to the code above. In the category 461, for example, the *exclude* note states that the category does not include chronic or unspecified sinusitis. The note may also give the code(s) of the excluded condition(s).

Excludes notes apply to the chapter, section, or category under which they appear. For example, the note *"Excludes that with heart involvement"* appears beneath category 390, Rheumatic fever without mention of heart involvement. If a diagnostic statement mentions rheumatic arthritis, rheumatic fever, or articular rheumatism and heart involvement, this category is inappropriate.

Colons in Includes and Excludes Notes

A colon (:) in an *includes* or *excludes* note indicates an incomplete term. One or more of the entries following the colon is required to make a complete term. Unlike terms in parentheses or brackets, when the colon is used, the diagnostic statement must include one of the terms after the colon to be assigned a code from the particular category. For example, the *excludes* note after the information for *coma* is as follows:

780.0 Alteration of consciousness

Excludes: coma:
diabetic (250.2–250.3)
    hepatic (572.2)
    originating in the perinatal period (779.2)

For the *excludes* note to apply to *coma*, "diabetic," " hepatic," or "originating in the perinatal period" must appear in the diagnostic statement.

Parentheses

Parentheses ( ) are used around descriptions that do not affect the code—that is, supplementary terms. For example, the subcategory 453.9, other venous embolism and thrombosis, of unspecified site, is followed by the entry "thrombosis (vein)."

Brackets

Brackets [ ] are used around synonyms, alternative wordings, or explanations. They have the same meaning as parentheses. For example, category 460, acute nasopharyngitis, is followed by the entry "[common cold]."

Braces

Braces } enclose a series of terms that are attached to the statement that appears to the right of the brace. They are an alternate format for a long list after a colon and also indicate incomplete terms. For example, the information after code 786.59, Chest pain, other, is as follows:

Discomfort ⎫
Pressure ⎬ in chest
Tightness ⎭

For this code to be applied to a diagnosis of "chest pain, other," "discomfort," "pressure," or "tightness" must appear in the statement.

Lozenge

The lozenge (◉) next to a code shows that it is not part of the World Health Organization's ICD. It appears only in the ICD-9-CM. This symbol can be ignored in coding diagnostic statements.

Abbreviations

NEC, not elsewhere classified, is found in the Tabular List as well as in the Alphabetic Index. Another abbreviation, NOS, or not otherwise specified, means unspecified. This term or abbreviation indicates that the code above it should be used when a condition is not completely described in the diagnostic statement or elsewhere in the patient medical record. For example, the code 827, other, multiple, and ill-defined fractures of lower limb, includes "leg NOS." If the documentation reads "patient suffered a fractured leg," this code is appropriate, since there is not enough information to determine which bone in the leg is involved. Note, however, that third-party payers may deny claims that use unspecified diagnosis codes. When possible, more-specific clinical documentation should be requested of the provider.

Multiple Codes

Some phrases contain instructions about the need for additional codes. The phrases point to situations in which more than one code is required to properly reflect the diagnostic statement. For example, a statement that a condition is "due to" or "associated with" may require an additional code.

Code First Underlying Disease

The instruction *code first underlying disease* appears below a code that must not be used as a primary code. These codes are for symptoms only, never for causes. The codes and their descriptions are in italic type, meaning that the code cannot be listed first even if the diagnostic statement is written that way. The phrase *code first associated disorder* or *code first underlying disorder* may appear below the italicized code and term. At times, a specific instruction is given, such as in this example:

366.31 Glaucomatous flecks (subcapsular)
      Code first underlying glaucoma (365.0–365.9)

Use Additional Code, Code Also, or Use Additional Code, if Desired

If a code is followed by the instruction *use an additional code* or *code also*, or a note saying the same thing, two codes are required. The order of the codes must be the same as shown in the Alphabetic Index: The etiology comes first, followed by the manifestation code.

The phrase *use additional code, if desired*, also means to use an additional code if it can be determined. This instruction may apply to an entire chapter, or it may appear in a subcategory following a code. When the diagnostic statement has sufficient information, an additional code is determined in the same way as *code first underlying disease*. For example, code 711.00, pyogenic arthritis (site unspecified), is followed by the phrase:

Use additional code, if desired, to identify infectious organisms (041.0–041.8)

In this case, if the documentation indicates it, the infectious organism causing the condition is coded.

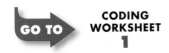

GO TO
CODING WORKSHEET 1

> *Note: The icon in the margin tells you to test your understanding at this point by completing a worksheet. Worksheets are located in Part 4 at the back of the text/workbook and are numbered consecutively. Coding Worksheet 1 is on pages 99–100.*

V CODES AND E CODES

Two supplementary classifications follow the chapters of the Tabular List:

- V codes identify encounters for reasons other than illness or injury.
- E codes identify the external causes of injuries and poisoning.

Both V and E codes are alphanumeric; they contain letters followed by numbers. For example, the code for a complete physical examination of an adult is V70.0. The code for a fall from a ladder is E881.0.

Using V Codes

V codes are used

- For visits with healthy patients who receive services other than treatments, such as annual checkups, immunizations, and normal childbirth. This use is coded by a V code that identifies the service, such as

  V06.4   Prophylactic vaccination/inoculation against measles-mumps-rubella (MMR)

- For visits with patients having known conditions for which they are receiving one of three types of treatment: chemotherapy, radiation therapy, and rehabilitation. In these cases, the encounter is coded first with a V code, and the condition is listed second. For example:

  V58.1   Encounter for chemotherapy

  233.0   Breast carcinoma

Listing the V code first for these three treatments is an exception to general coding rules. Usually, when patients receive therapeutic treatments for already diagnosed conditions, the previously diagnosed condition is used for the primary code.

- For visits in which a problem not currently affecting the patient's health status needs to be noted. For example, codes V10–V19 cover history. If a person with a family history of colon cancer presents with rectal bleeding, the problem is listed first, and the V code is assigned as an additional code, as is shown here:

569.3   Hemorrhage of rectum and anus

V16.0   Family history of malignant neoplasm

- For visits in which patients are being evaluated preoperatively, a code from category V72.8 is listed first, followed by a code for the condition that is the reason for the surgery. For example:

V72.81   Preoperative cardiovascular examination

414.01   Arteriosclerotic heart disease of native coronary artery

A V code can be used as either a primary code for an encounter or as an additional code. It is looked up in the same way as other codes, using the Alphabetic Index to find the term's code and the Supplementary Classification in the Tabular List to verify it. The terms that indicate the need for V codes, however, are not the same as other medical terms. They usually have to do with a reason for an encounter other than a disease or its complications. When found in diagnostic statements, the words listed in the first column of Table 1.2 often point to V codes.

TABLE 1.2   Terminology Associated with V Codes

TERMS	V CODE	EXAMPLE
Contact	V01.1	Contact with tuberculosis
Contraception	V25.1	Insertion of intrauterine contraceptive device
Counseling	V61.11	Counseling for victim of spousal and partner abuse
Examination	V70	General medical examination
Fitting of	V52	Fitting and adjustment of prosthetic device and implant
Follow-up	V67.0	Follow-up examination following surgery
Health or healthy	V20	Health supervision of infant or child
History (of)	V10.05	Personal history of malignant neoplasm, large intestine
Replacement	V42.0	Kidney replaced by transplant
Screening/test	V73.2	Special screening examination for measles
Status	V44	Artificial opening status
Supervision (of)	V23	Supervision of high-risk pregnancy
Therapy	V57.3	Speech therapy
Vaccination/inoculation	V06	Need for prophylactic vaccination and inoculation against combinations of disease

Using E Codes

E (for external) codes classify injuries resulting from environmental events such as falls, fires, transportation accidents, accidental poisoning by a drug or other substances, and **adverse effects**, which are a patient's harmful reaction to the correct dosage of a drug (categories E930 to E949).

The Table of Drugs and Chemicals that appears after the Alphabetic Index lists these agents alphabetically, and columns 2 through 6 contain the E codes for the situation: accidental, therapeutic, suicide attempt, assault, or undetermined use of the drug or chemical. The Alphabetic Index to External Causes of Injury and Poisoning that follows the Table of Drugs and Chemicals lists main terms for external causes, describing the accident, circumstance, event, or specific agent (drug or chemical) that caused the injury.

E codes are located by first using the Alphabetic Index to External Causes of Injury and Poisoning and verifying the code assignment in the Supplementary Classifications section of the Tabular List.

> **Coding Point**
>
> **E Codes—A Supplementary Classification**
> External causes are not the primary diagnoses of patients' conditions, so E codes are never used alone. Instead, E codes always supplement a code that identifies the injury or condition itself. The primary diagnosis code is listed first, followed by the additional E code.

E codes are often used in collecting public health information. These categories are important in medical practices:

- *Accidents:* When patients have accidents, payers check the E codes that are assigned to verify that the services are covered by the medical insurance policy, rather than by an automobile policy or workers' compensation laws.

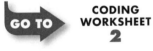
CODING WORKSHEET 2

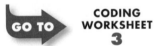
CODING WORKSHEET 3

- *Drug reactions:* The categories E930 to E949 apply to a patient's unintentional, harmful reaction to a proper dosage of a drug–adverse effects. The specific drug is located in the Table of Drugs and Chemicals in the Alphabetic Index. Adverse effects are different from poisoning, which refers to the medical result of the incorrect use of a substance. Poisoning codes are found under categories 960–979.

CODING STEPS

The correct procedure for reporting accurate diagnosis codes has three steps.

Step 1 Analyze the Reason for the Encounter

The first step is to identify the diagnosis that is to be coded. The diagnosis is usually based on the patient's chief complaint and the physician's findings. To find the diagnosis, the coder works with the documentation of the patient's encounter. In some situations, this documentation may be brief, such as the physician's statement of the diagnosis on an encounter form. In other cases, the coder works with a complex medical record, such as progress reports, operative reports, or histories.

If there is more than one condition or complaint, the **primary diagnosis**, the main reason for the patient encounter, must be determined. The primary diagnosis is the diagnosis, condition, problem, or other reason that the documentation shows as being chiefly responsible for the services that are provided.

Step 2 Apply the Appropriate Coding Guidelines

The primary diagnosis for the encounter provides the main term to be coded first. If other conditions or problems are pertinent, they are also coded. Coders apply the appropriate guidelines, such as using five-digit codes when possible.

> **Coding Point**
>
> **Outpatient versus Inpatient Diagnoses**
> Note that physician practice coding uses a different rule than hospital (inpatient) coding. In the inpatient setting, the reason the patient has been admitted is called the principal (rather than primary) diagnosis, and often it is not known until the end of the hospital stay.

Step 3 Assign the Code

To assign the code, first locate the main term for the patient's primary diagnosis in the Alphabetic Index. Follow these steps:

- Use any supplementary terms in the diagnostic statement to help locate the main term.
- Read and follow any notes below the main term.
- Review the subterms to find the most specific match to the diagnosis.
- Read and follow any cross-references.
- Make note of a two-code (etiology and/or manifestation) indication.

Then, verify the code for the main term in the Tabular List:

- Read *includes* or *excludes* notes, checking back to see if any apply to the code's category, section, or chapter.
- Be alert for and observe fifth-digit requirements.
- Follow any instructions requiring the selection of additional codes (such as "code also" or "code first underlying disease").
- List multiple codes in the correct order.

> **Coding Point**
>
> **Correct Coding Procedure**
> Never use only the Alphabetic Index or only the Tabular List to code. Either practice causes coding errors.

KEY CODING GUIDELINES

Diagnostic coding in medical practices follows specific guidelines. These are developed by a group made up of CMS advisers and participants from the American Hospital Association, the American Health Information Management Association, and the National Center for Health Statistics.

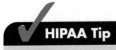

HIPAA Tip

AHA CODING CLINIC
The official guidelines for ICD-9-CM coding are published quarterly in the American Hospital Association's *Coding Clinic.*

As illustrated in Figure 1.3, the guidelines cover all the rules for what is to be coded and in what order the codes should be listed. In this section, three key guidelines are discussed:

1. Code the primary diagnosis first, followed by current coexisting conditions.
2. Code to the highest level of certainty.
3. Code to the highest level of specificity.

Diagnostic Coding and Reporting Guidelines for Outpatient Services

These coding guidelines for outpatient diagnoses have been approved for use by hospitals/ physicians in coding and reporting hospital-based outpatient services and physician office visits.

Information about the use of certain abbreviations, punctuation, symbols, and other conventions used in the ICD-9-CM Tabular List (code numbers and titles), can be found in Section IA of these guidelines, under "Conventions Used in the Tabular List." Information about the correct sequence to use in finding a code is also described in Section I.

The terms encounter and visit are often used interchangeably in describing outpatient service contacts and, therefore, appear together in these guidelines without distinguishing one from the other.

Though the conventions and general guidelines apply to all settings, coding guidelines for outpatient and physician reporting of diagnoses will vary in a number of instances from those for inpatient diagnoses, recognizing that:

The Uniform Hospital Discharge Data Set (UHDDS) definition of principal diagnosis applies only to inpatients in acute, short-term, general hospitals.

Coding guidelines for inconclusive diagnoses (probable, suspected, rule out, etc.) were developed for inpatient reporting and do not apply to outpatients.

A. Selection of first-listed condition

   In the outpatient setting, the term first-listed diagnosis is used in lieu of principal diagnosis.

   In determining the first-listed diagnosis the coding conventions of ICD-9-CM, as well as the general and disease specific guidelines take precedence over the outpatient guidelines.

   Diagnoses often are not established at the time of the initial encounter/visit. It may take two or more visits before the diagnosis is confirmed.

   The most critical rule involves beginning the search for the correct code assignment through the Alphabetic Index. Never begin searching initially in the Tabular List as this will lead to coding errors.

B. The appropriate code or codes from 001.0 through V83.89 must be used to identify diagnoses, symptoms, conditions, problems, complaints, or other reason(s) for the encounter/visit.

C. For accurate reporting of ICD-9-CM diagnosis codes, the documentation should describe the patient's condition, using terminology which includes specific diagnoses as well as symptoms, problems, or reasons for the encounter. There are ICD-9-CM codes to describe all of these.

D. The selection of codes 001.0 through 999.9 will frequently be used to describe the reason for the encounter. These codes are from the section of ICD-9-CM for the classification of diseases and injuries (e.g. infectious and parasitic diseases; neoplasms; symptoms, signs, and ill-defined conditions, etc.).

E. Codes that describe symptoms and signs, as opposed to diagnoses, are acceptable for reporting purposes when a diagnosis has not been established (confirmed) by the physician. Chapter 16 of ICD-9-CM, Symptoms, Signs, and Ill-defined conditions (codes 780.0 - 799.9) contain many, but not all codes for symptoms.

F. ICD-9-CM provides codes to deal with encounters for circumstances other than a disease or injury. The Supplementary Classification of factors Influencing Health Status and Contact with Health Services (VO1.0- V83.89) is provided to deal with occasions when circumstances other than a disease or injury are recorded as diagnosis or problems.

FIGURE 1.3 ICD-9-CM Guidelines for Coding and Reporting Outpatient Services

G. Level of Detail in Coding

    1. ICD-9-CM is composed of codes with either 3, 4, or 5 digits. Codes with three digits are included in ICD-9-CM as the heading of a category of codes that may be further subdivided by the use of fourth and/or fifth digits, which provide greater specificity.

    2. A three-digit code is to be used only if it is not further subdivided. Where fourth-digit subcategories and/or fifth-digit subclassifications are provided, they must be assigned. A code is invalid if it has not been coded to the full number of digits required for that code. See also discussion under Section I, General Coding Guidelines, Level of Detail.

H. List first the ICD-9-CM code for the diagnosis, condition, problem, or other reason for encounter/visit shown in the medical record to be chiefly responsible for the services provided. List additional codes that describe any coexisting conditions.

I. Do not code diagnoses documented as "probable," "suspected," "questionable," "rule out," or "working diagnosis." Rather, code the condition(s) to the highest degree of certainty for that encounter/visit, such as symptoms, signs, abnormal test results, or other reason for the visit.

Please note: This differs from the coding practices used by hospital medical record departments for coding the diagnosis of acute care, short-term hospital inpatients.

J. Chronic diseases treated on an ongoing basis may be coded and reported as many times as the patient receives treatment and care for the condition(s).

K. Code all documented conditions that coexist at the time of the encounter/visit, and require or affect patient care treatment or management. Do not code conditions that were previously treated and no longer exist. However, history codes (VIO-V19) may be used as secondary codes if the historical condition or family history has an impact on current care or influences treatment.

L. For patients receiving diagnostic services only during an encounter/visit, sequence first the diagnosis, condition, problem, or other reason for encounter/visit shown in the medical record to be chiefly responsible for the outpatient services provided during the encounter/visit. Codes for other diagnoses (e.g., chronic conditions) may be sequenced as additional diagnoses.

For outpatient encounters for diagnostic tests that have been interpreted by a physician, and the final report is available at the time of coding, code any confirmed or definitive diagnosis(es) documented in the interpretation. Do not code related signs and symptoms as additional diagnoses.

Please note: This differs from the coding practice in the hospital inpatient setting regarding abnormal findings on test results.

M. For patients receiving therapeutic services only during an encounter/visit, sequence first the diagnosis, condition, problem, or other reason for encounter/visit shown in the medical record to be chiefly responsible for the outpatient services provided during the encounter/visit. Codes for other diagnoses (e.g., chronic conditions) may be sequenced as additional diagnoses.

The only exception to this rule is that when the primary reason for the admission/encounter is chemotherapy, radiation therapy, or rehabilitation, the appropriate V code for the service is listed first, and the diagnosis or problem for which the service is being performed listed second.

N. For patients receiving preoperative evaluations only, sequence a code from category V72.8, Other specified examinations, to describe the pre-op consultations. Assign a code for the condition to describe the reason for the surgery as an additional diagnosis. Code also any findings related to the pre-op evaluation.

O. For ambulatory surgery, code the diagnosis for which the surgery was performed. If the postoperative diagnosis is known to be different from the preoperative diagnosis at the time the diagnosis is confirmed, select the postoperative diagnosis for coding, since it is the most definitive.

P. For routine outpatient prenatal visits when no complications are present codes V22.0, Supervision of normal first pregnancy, and V22.l, Supervision of other normal pregnancy, should be used as principal diagnoses. These codes should not be used in conjunction with chapter 11 codes.

FIGURE 1.3 ICD-9-CM Guidelines for Coding and Reporting Outpatient Services, *continued*

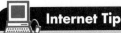
Code the Primary Diagnosis First, Followed by Current Coexisting Conditions

The ICD-9-CM code for the primary diagnosis is listed first.

Example

Diagnostic Statement: Patient is an elderly female complaining of back pain. For the past five days, she has had signs of pyelonephritis, including urinary urgency, urinary incontinence, and back pain. Has had a little hematuria, but no past history of urinary difficulties.

Primary Diagnosis: 590.80   Pyelonephritis

Additional codes are listed to describe all current documented coexisting conditions—conditions that affect patient treatment or require treatment during the encounter. Coexisting conditions may be related to the primary diagnosis, or they may involve a separate illness that the physician diagnoses and treats during the encounter.

Example

Diagnostic Statement: Patient, a forty-five-year-old male, presents for complete physical examination for an insurance certification. During the examination, patient complains of occasional difficulty hearing; wax is removed from the left ear canal.

Primary Diagnosis: V70.3   Routine physical examination for insurance certification

Coexisting Condition: 380.4   Impacted cerumen

It is important to note that patients may have diseases or conditions that do not affect the encounter being coded. Some physicians add notes about previous conditions to provide an easy reference to a patient's history. Unless these conditions are directly involved with the patient's treatment, they are not considered in selecting codes. Also, conditions that were previously treated and no longer exist are not coded.

Example

Chart Note: Mrs. Mackenzie, whose previous encounter was for her regularly scheduled blood pressure check, presents today with a new onset of psoriasis.

Primary Diagnosis: 696.1   Psoriasis, NOS

If the reason for the visit is a condition other than a disease or illness, the appropriate V code is used to code the encounter:

Example

V72.3   Routine gynecological examination with Papanicolaou smear

Coding Acute versus Chronic Conditions

The reasons for patient encounters are often **acute** symptoms—generally, relatively sudden or severe problems. Acute conditions are coded with the specific code that is designated acute, if listed. Many patients, however, receive ongoing treatment for **chronic** conditions—those that continue over a long period of time or recur frequently. For example, a patient may need a regular gold injection for the management of rheumatoid arthritis. In such cases, the disease is coded and reported for as many times as the patient receives care for the condition.

In some cases, an encounter covers both an acute and a chronic condition. Some conditions do not have separate entries for both manifestations, so a single code applies. If both the acute and the chronic illnesses have codes, the acute code is listed first.

Example

Acute Renal Failure   584.9

Chronic Renal Failure   585

Coding Late Effects

A **late effect** is a condition that remains after a patient's acute illness or injury has ended. Often called residual effects, some late effects happen soon after the disease is over, and others occur later. The diagnostic statement may say "late, due to an old . . ."or "due to a previous . . . ." In general, the main term *late* is followed by subterms that list the causes. Two codes are usually required. First reported is the code for the specific late effect (such as muscle soreness), followed by the code for the cause of the late effect (such as the late effect of rickets).

Code to the Highest Level of Certainty

If the physician has not established a diagnosis, the diagnosis codes that cover symptoms, signs, and ill-defined conditions are used. Inconclusive diagnoses, such as those preceded by "rule out," "suspected," or "probable," for example, are not coded. This rule—code only to the highest degree of certainty—exists because an unproven condition reported to a payer could prove damaging to the patient; such a statement could remain in others' records uncorrected. For example, if the diagnostic statement said "rule out aggressive breast carcinoma," a code for that disease was used, and a malignancy was not found, the patient could be denied medical insurance coverage because of the insurer's concern that the patient has cancer.

Coding Signs and Symptoms

Diagnoses are not always established at the first encounter. Two or more visits may be required before the physician determines a primary diagnosis. During this process, although possible diagnoses may appear in a patient's medical record as the physician's work is progressing, these inconclusive diagnoses are not reported for reimbursement of service fees. Instead, the specific signs and symptoms are coded and reported. A *sign* is an objective indication that can be evaluated by the physician, such as weight loss. A *symptom* is a subjective statement by the patient that cannot be confirmed during an examination, such as pain. The following case provides an example of how symptoms and signs are coded:

Example

Diagnostic Statement: Middle-aged male presents with abdominal pain and weight loss. He had to return home from vacation because he was too ill. He has not been eating well because of a vague upper-abdominal pain. He denies nausea, vomiting. He denies changes in bowel habit or blood in stool. Physical examination revealed no abdominal tenderness.

Primary Diagnosis: 789.06   Abdominal pain, epigastric region

Coexisting Condition: 783.2   Abnormal loss of weight

Coding the Reason for Surgery

Surgery is coded according to the diagnosis that is listed as the reason for the procedure. In some cases, the postoperative diagnosis is available and is different from the physician's primary diagnosis before the surgery. If so, the postoperative diagnosis is coded because it is the highest level of certainty available. For example, if an excisional biopsy is performed to evaluate mammographic breast lesions or a lump of unknown nature, and the pathology results show a malignant neoplasm, the diagnosis code describing the site and nature of the neoplasm is used. (Coding neoplasms is covered later in this chapter.)

Code to the Highest Level of Specificity

A three-digit code is used only if a four-digit code is not provided in the ICD-9-CM. Likewise, a four-digit subcategory code is used only when no five-digit subclassification is listed. When a five-digit code is available, it must be used.

The more digits the code has, the more specific it becomes; the additional codes add to the clinical picture of the patient. Using the most specific code possible is referred to as coding to the highest level of specificity.

Example

The category code 250 indicates a diagnosis of diabetes mellitus. Under this category, a fourth digit provides information about the cause or site, such as

250.1   Diabetes with ketoacidosis

250.2   Diabetes with hyperosmolarity

250.3   Diabetes with other coma

250.4   Diabetes with renal manifestations

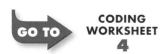

GO TO CODING WORKSHEET **4**

A fifth digit must be added to any of these four-digit codes, according to which of these is documented:

0   Type II or unspecified type, not stated as uncontrolled
1   Type I, not stated as uncontrolled
2   Type II or unspecified type, uncontrolled
3   Type I, uncontrolled

Type I is insulin-dependent; type II is not. *Control* indicates whether the glycemic level (blood sugar) is under control. An uncontrolled diabetic is likely to become blind, lose limbs through amputation because of severely reduced circulation, and experience renal failure. On the other hand, a controlled diabetic usually leads a substantially normal life. The diagnostic code 250.33 indicates diabetes mellitus with other coma, insulin-dependent, and uncontrolled. This diagnosis presents a very different clinical picture than 250.40, diabetes mellitus with renal manifestations, not insulin-dependent, and not stated as being uncontrolled.

CODING PRACTICE

Accurate assignment of ICD codes requires practice! In the following pages, each chapter of the ICD-9-CM is briefly introduced. Any special guidelines needed to accurately code are then described. After studying this material, you will complete worksheets to apply your knowledge of the diagnosis codes for the ICD chapter. Some worksheets have coding points to help you assign the correct ICD codes.

Infectious and Parasitic Diseases— Codes 001–139

Codes in Chapter 1 of the ICD-9-CM's Tabular List classify communicable infectious and parasitic diseases. Most categories describe a condition and the type of organism that causes it. For example, category 004, shigellosis, describes acute infectious dysentery caused by Shigella bacteria. This category's codes classify four groups of bacteria plus a code for other *specified* Shigella infections, which occur infrequently, and a code for *unspecified* shigellosis for use when the condition is insufficiently described in the medical documentation for specific code assignment.

Note that in the Tabular List, the word *includes* followed by descriptions of conditions helps the coder confirm the correct classification. These notes apply to the chapter, section, or category under which they appear. For example, the note *"Includes infection or food poisoning by Salmonella"* appears beneath category 003, Other salmonella infections, and applies to infection or food poisoning caused by any organism in the category—that is, all the codes that begin with 003.

GO TO CODING WORKSHEET **5**

Neoplasms— Codes 140–239

Neoplasms are coded from Chapter 2 of the ICD-9-CM. Neoplasms, also called tumors, are growths that arise from normal tissue. Note that this category does not include a diagnosis statement with the word *mass*, which is a separate main term.

The Neoplasm Table

The Alphabetic Index contains a Neoplasm Table that points to codes for neoplasms. The table lists the anatomical location in the first column. The next six columns relate to the behavior of the neoplasm, described as

- One of the following three types of malignant tumor, each of which is progressive, rapid-growing, life-threatening, and made of cancerous cells:

  Primary: The neoplasm that is the encounter's main diagnosis is found at the site of origin.

  Secondary: The neoplasm that is the encounter's main diagnosis metastasized (spread) to an additional body site from the original location.

  Carcinoma in situ: The neoplasm is restricted to one site (a noninvasive type); this may also be referred to as *preinvasive cancer.*

- Benign—slow-growing, not life-threatening, made of normal or near-normal cells
- Uncertain behavior—not classifiable when the cells were examined
- Unspecified nature—no documentation of the nature of the neoplasm.

As an example, the following entries are shown in the Neoplasm Table for a neoplasm of the colon:

	MALIGNANT					
	Primary	Secondary	Cancer in situ	BENIGN	UNCERTAIN BEHAVIOR	UNSPECIFIED
Colon	154.0	197.5	230.4	211.4	235.2	239.0

Note that in physician coding, you avoid reporting suspected or possible conditions. Before pathology work identifies the behavior of a tumor, the condition can be classified with a code in the range 780–799 (Symptoms, Signs, or Ill-Defined Conditions), if applicable, or with V71.1 (observation for suspected malignant neoplasm, not found) or V76 (screening for malignant neoplasms).

In the Tabular List, neoplasms are listed in Chapter 2 under categories 140 to 239.

M Codes

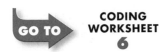

GO TO
CODING WORKSHEET 6

In the regular Alphabetic Index entries, the pointers for neoplasms also show morphology codes, known as M codes. M codes contain the letter M followed by four digits, a slash, and a final digit. M codes (listed in ICD-9-CM, Appendix A) are used by pathologists to report on and study the prevalence of various types of neoplasms. They are not used in physician practice (outpatient) coding.

Endocrine, Nutritional, and Metabolic Diseases, and Immunity Disorders—Codes 240–279

Codes in Chapter 3 of the ICD-9-CM classify a variety of conditions. The most common disease in Chapter 3 is diabetes mellitus, which is a progressive disease of either type I or type II. Ninety percent of cases are type II.

In type I (category I) diabetes, the patient's health depends on receiving regular insulin injections and following a strict regimen to avoid serious complications. Type I may also be called juvenile type or juvenile onset, because most cases appear before age 30. In type II (category II), the patient's condition may be managed with medication, diet, and exercise, although a requirement for insulin may occur. Type II may also be called adult onset or maturity onset.

Another common condition is obesity, in which body weight is beyond skeletal and physical requirements because of excessive accumulation of body fat. Obesity is associated with a number of primary conditions, such as coronary artery disease, gall bladder disease, high cholesterol, hypertension, and type II diabetes mellitus.

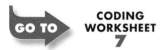

GO TO CODING WORKSHEET 7

Diseases of the Blood and Blood-Forming Organs—Codes 280–289

Codes in this brief ICD-9-CM chapter (Chapter 4) classify diseases of the blood and blood-forming organs, such as anemia and coagulation defects.

As you practice coding skills in this ICD-9-CM chapter, remember that:

- Two punctuation marks—the colon and the brace—are used in the Tabular List of the ICD-9-CM to introduce diagnostic terms that are connected to the term they follow. These modifying terms help the coder verify the correct code. For example, under subcategory 281.0 Pernicious anemia, the terms *Addison's*, *Biermer's*, and *congenital pernicious* each modify the term *anemia*.

- NEC and NOS have different meanings and uses. NEC stands for Not Elsewhere Classified. This abbreviation appears with a term when there is no code that is specific for the condition. It means that no code matches the particular problem described in the diagnostic statement. In this case, the coder has specific documentation, but ICD-9-CM does not provide a code that matches the statement. NOS, which stands for Not Otherwise Specified, means that the diagnostic statement does not provide enough information to classify the condition.

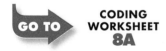

GO TO CODING WORKSHEET 8A

Mental Disorders— Codes 290–319

Codes in Chapter 5 of the ICD-9-CM classify the various types of mental disorders, including conditions of drug and alcohol dependency, Alzheimer's disease, schizophrenic disorders, and mood disturbances.

Most psychiatrists use the terminology found in the *Diagnostic and Statistical Manual of Mental Disorders (DSM)* for diagnoses, but the coding

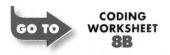

GO TO CODING WORKSHEET **8B**

follows the ICD-9-CM. Appendix B of the ICD-9-CM contains a glossary of mental disorders. These psychiatric terms are used by physicians in diagnostic statements. This reference may be helpful in determining correct codes in the Mental Disorders chapter.

Diseases of the Nervous System and Sense Organs—Codes 320–389

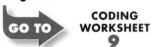

GO TO CODING WORKSHEET **9**

Codes in Chapter 6 classify diseases of the central nervous system, the peripheral nervous system, the eye, and the ear.

Diseases of the Circulatory System— Codes 390–459

Because the circulatory system involves so many interrelated components, the disease process can create interrelated, complex conditions. Many types of cardiovascular system disease, such as acute myocardial infarction (heart attack), require hospitalization of patients. The following introduction covers some frequently coded diagnoses. The notes and *code also* instructions in Chapter 7 of the Tabular List must be carefully observed to code circulatory diseases accurately.

Ischemic Heart Disease and Arteriosclerotic Cardiovascular Disease

Ischemic heart disease conditions—those caused by reduced blood flow to the heart—are coded under categories 410 to 414. Myocardial infarctions that are acute or have a documented duration of eight weeks or less are located in category 410. Chronic myocardial infarctions, or those with duration longer than eight weeks, are coded to subcategory 414.8. An old or healed myocardial infarction without current symptoms is coded 412.

Other chronic ischemic heart diseases are coded under category 414. Coronary atherosclerosis, 414.0, requires a fifth digit for the type of artery involved and includes arteriosclerotic heart disease (ASHD), atherosclerotic heart disease, and other coronary conditions. A diagnosis of angina pectoris—an episode of chest pain from a temporary insufficiency of oxygen to the heart—is coded 413.9, unless it occurs only at night (413.0) or is diagnosed as Prinzmetal (angiospastic) angina (413.1).

Arteriosclerotic cardiovascular disease (ASCVD)—hardening of the arteries affecting the complete cardiovascular system—is coded 429.2. A second code for the arteriosclerosis, 440.9, is also needed for this diagnosis. Likewise, 440.9 is never the primary code when ASCVD is a diagnosis.

Hypertension and Hypertensive Heart Disease

Hypertension is a diagnosis related to high blood pressure. Almost all cases are due to unknown causes. This is called essential hypertension and is the primary diagnosis. In the few cases where the cause is known, the hypertension is called secondary, and its code is listed after the code for the cause.

Within the essential hypertension category, there are three subcategories: malignant (401.0), benign (401.1), and unspecified (401.9). Malignant hypertension is an extremely serious condition, so it is always documented as malignant. Benign hypertension is a relatively mild and often chronic condition. If the diagnostic statement does not contain either word, the hypertension is coded as unspecified. Hypertension can affect the heart and/or the kidneys. Hypertensive heart disease and hypertensive renal disease are coded under the categories 402 to 404.

Note that a diagnosis of hypertension is different from "high (or elevated) blood pressure." If the diagnosis does not include *hypertension*, the statement is coded 796.2, elevated blood pressure reading without diagnosis of hypertension (from the Symptoms, Signs, and Ill-Defined Conditions chapter of the ICD-9-CM).

The Alphabetic Index contains a detailed table to point to the various types of hypertensive disease, including its effect on pregnancy. Hypertension is often indicated as a coexisting condition with other conditions, and it may make those more serious. When these diagnoses appear, two codes must be assigned, one for the first condition and one for the hypertension.

Example

Diagnosis of angina pectoris with essential hypertension: 413.9 and 401.9

CODING WORKSHEET 10

Diseases of the Respiratory System— Codes 460–519

CODING WORKSHEET 11

Codes in Chapter 8 of the ICD-9-CM classify respiratory illnesses such as pneumonia, chronic obstructive pulmonary disease (COPD), and asthma. Pneumonia, a common respiratory infection, may be caused by one of a number of organisms. Many codes for pneumonia include the condition and the cause in a combination code, such as 480.2, pneumonia due to parainfluenza virus.

Diseases of the Digestive System— Codes 520–579

CODING WORKSHEET 12

Codes in Chapter 9 of the ICD-9-CM classify diseases of the digestive system. Codes are listed according to anatomical location, beginning with the oral cavity and continuing through the intestines.

Diseases of the Genitourinary System— Codes 580–629

CODING WORKSHEET 13

Codes in Chapter 10 of the ICD-9-CM classify diseases of the male and female genitourinary (GU) systems, such as infections of the genital tract, renal disease, conditions of the prostate, and problems with the cervix, vulva, and breast.

Complications of Pregnancy, Childbirth, and the Puerperium— Codes 630–677

GO TO CODING WORKSHEET 14

Codes in Chapter 11 of the ICD-9-CM classify conditions that are involved with pregnancy, childbirth, and the puerperium (the six-week period following delivery). Many categories require a fifth digit that is based on when the complications occur (referred to as the episode of care), either before birth (antepartum), during, or after birth (postpartum). Valid fifth digits are usually shown in brackets next to the subcategory.

Note that codes in this chapter refer only to conditions of the *mother*, not of the infant. They cover the course of pregnancy and childbirth from conception through the puerperium. Codes for conditions that affect newborns are in ICD-9-CM's Chapter 15.

Diseases of the Skin and Subcutaneous Tissue— Codes 680–709

GO TO CODING WORKSHEET 15

Codes in the ICD-9-CM's Chapter 12 classify skin infections, inflammations, and other diseases.

Coders should be aware that an entire chapter or section may be subject to "Excludes" or "Includes" notes, based on the note's location. For example, the first section in this chapter (680–686) begins with a note excluding certain skin infections that are classified in Chapter 1.

Diseases of the Musculoskeletal System and Connective Tissue— Codes 710–739

GO TO CODING WORKSHEET 16

Codes in Chapter 12 of the ICD-9-CM classify conditions of the bones and joints—arthropathies (joint disorders), dorsopathies (back disorders), rheumatism, and other diseases. The chapter opens with a description of the fifth digits to be used for many categories. The subclassifications are organized by body site, from unspecified to multiple. The list also identifies the bones and joints that are included in each fifth digit. Remember to refer to this master list, because later in the chapter this subclassification appears in shortened form before the category and in brackets next to the code and description.

Congenital Anomalies— Codes 740–759

GO TO CODING WORKSHEET 17A

Codes in this brief ICD-9-CM Chapter 14 classify anomalies, malformations, and diseases that exist at birth. Unlike acquired disorders, congenital conditions are either hereditary or due to influencing factors during gestation.

Although congenital anomalies are defined as existing at birth, they do not always immediately affect the patient. As examples, normal human beings have 33 vertebrae, but a person without the normal number may be asymptomatic, and patients with dominant polycystic disease may not experience impaired function until adulthood. The classifications for congenital anomalies thus are not related to patients' ages.

Certain Conditions Originating in the Perinatal Period— Codes 760–779

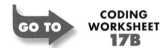

Codes in Chapter 15 of the ICD-9-CM classify conditions of the fetus or the newborn infant, the neonate, up to 28 days after birth. These codes are assigned only to conditions of the infant, not of the mother. (Codes for conditions that affect the management of the mother's pregnancy are in Chapter 11.) They cover the perinatal period, which is the period from shortly before birth until 28 days following delivery. When the hospitalization that results in the birth is to be coded, these codes are secondary to codes from categories V30 through V39. Note the use of the fourth digit to designate the birth location and of the fifth digit to specify hospital births.

Symptoms, Signs, and Ill-Defined Conditions— Codes 780–799

Codes in this sixteenth chapter of the ICD-9-CM classify patients' signs, symptoms, and ill-defined conditions for which a definitive diagnosis cannot be made. In physician practice coding, these codes are always used instead of coding "rule out," "probable," or "suspected" conditions.

High Blood Pressure

High (or elevated) blood pressure is coded as 796.2, "elevated blood pressure reading without diagnosis of hypertension." This diagnosis is not the same as hypertension, as coded in Chapter 7 for diseases of the circulatory system.

HIV/AIDS Codes

HIV coding is complex. When a diagnosis of HIV infection has been made, code 042 is used to classify any of the many terms used for this condition, such as AIDS, acquired immunodeficiency syndrome, and HIV disease. When a patient with no related symptoms has a screening test for HIV infection, code V73.89 is used. If the test results are positive for HIV infection but the patient shows no symptoms, code V08 is used. If, however, the test result is reported as "nonspecific serologic evidence of HIV," code 795.71 is used.

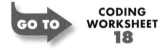

Injury and Poisoning— Codes 800–999

Codes in Chapter 17 of the ICD-9-CM classify injuries and wounds such as fractures, dislocations, sprains, strains, internal injuries, burns, and traumatic injuries. The chapter also includes a section covering poisoning and a section for the late effects of injuries and poisoning. Often, E codes are also used to identify the cause of the injury or poisoning.

Fractures

Fractures are coded using categories 800 to 829. A fourth digit indicates whether the fracture is closed or open. When a fracture is closed, the broken bone does not pierce the skin. An open fracture involves breaking through the skin. If the fracture is not indicated as open or closed, it is coded as closed. A fifth digit is often used for the specific anatomical site. For example:

810 Fracture of clavicle

The following fifth-digit subclassification is for use with category 810:

0   unspecified part (Clavicle NOS)
1   sternal end of clavicle
2   shaft of clavicle
3   acromial end of clavicle

⑤ **810.0 Closed**

⑤ **810.1 Open**

When any of the following descriptions are used, a closed fracture is indicated:

Comminuted	Greenstick	Simple
Depressed	Impacted	Slipped epiphysis
Elevated	Linear	Spiral
Fissured	March	Unspecified

These descriptions indicate open fractures:

Compound	Missile	With foreign body
Infected	Puncture	

Burns

Burns are located in categories 940 to 949, where they are classified according to the cause, such as flames or radiation. They are grouped by severity and by how much of the body's surface is involved. Severity is rated as one of three degrees of burns:

1. *First-degree burn:* The epidermis (outer layer of skin) is damaged.

2. *Second-degree burn:* Both the epidermis and the dermis are damaged.

3. *Third-degree burn:* The most severe degree; the three layers of the skin—epidermis, dermis, and subcutaneous—are all damaged.

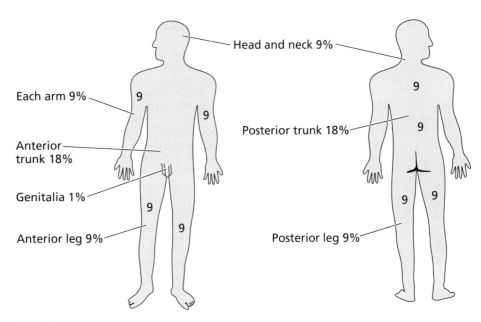

FIGURE 1.4 Coding Burns

The total body surface area (TBSA) that is involved determines the extent of the burn for coding purposes (see Figure 1.4). When burns are coded according to extent (category 948), fourth-digit codes are used to show the percentage of TBSA for all of the burns. For third-degree burns, a fifth digit is also required to classify the percentage of third-degree burns:

0   less than 10% or unspecified

1   10%–19%

2   20%–29%

3   30%–39%

4   40%–49%

5   50%–59%

6   60%–69%

7   70%–79%

8   80%–89%

9   90% or more of body surface

Poisoning versus Adverse Effects

Poisoning refers to the medical result of the incorrect use of a substance. This is different from accidental harm caused by an adverse effect due to reaction to the correct dosage of a drug. The Table of Drugs and Chemicals following the Alphabetic Index lists these agents alphabetically, and Column 1 contains the code for the poisoning. Use the Table first to point to a code that you verify in the Tabular List under categories 960–979.

Late Effects

Late, or residual, effects may occur soon after the acute phase or later in life. Late effects are indicated by expressions such as "late," "due to an old. . ." or "due to a previous. . ." followed by the cause. Check late effects in the Alphabetic Index for the location of the applicable code. Two codes are required. Code the specific residual (late) effect first, then list the code for its cause.

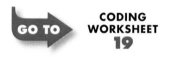

GO TO **CODING WORKSHEET 19**

CODING QUIZZES

The Coding Quizzes help you test your coding ability and practice your skills in working through certification examinations. You are ready to take the ICD Coding Quiz!

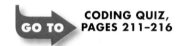

GO TO **CODING QUIZ, PAGES 211–216**

SUMMARY

1. The ICD-9-CM is the *Clinical Modification* of the World Health Organization's *International Classification of Diseases* used for diagnostic coding in the United States. ICD-9-CM codes are required for reporting patients' conditions on insurance claims and encounter forms. Codes are made up of three, four, or five numbers and a description. The addenda, which are lists of new, changed, or deleted codes, are issued annually. Medical practices must use the current codes because they can affect billing and reimbursement.

2. The ICD-9-CM has two volumes that are used in medical practices, the Tabular List (Volume 1) and the Alphabetic Index (Volume 2). The Alphabetic Index is used first in the process of finding a code. It contains an index of all the diseases that are classified in the Tabular List. These main terms may be followed by related subterms or supported by supplementary terms. The codes themselves are organized into seventeen chapters according to etiology or body system and are listed in numerical order in the Tabular List. Code categories consist of three-digit groupings of a single disease or a related condition. Subcategories have four digits to show the disease's etiology, site, or manifestation. Further clinical detail is supplied by fifth-digit subclassifications.

3. The conventions used in the ICD-9-CM must be observed to correctly select codes. Notes provide details about conditions that are either excluded or included under the code. The cross-reference *see* means that another main term is appropriate. A symbol is used to show a fifth-digit requirement. The abbreviation NOS (not otherwise specified or unspecified) indicates the code to use when a condition is not completely described. The abbreviation NEC (not elsewhere classified) indicates the code to use when the diagnosis does not match any other available code. Parentheses and brackets indicate supplementary terms. Colons and braces indicate that one or more words after the punctuation must appear in the diagnostic statement for the code to be applicable. Codes that are not used as primary appear in italics and are usually followed by an instruction to code first underlying disease or use additional code.

4. V codes identify encounters for reasons other than illness or injury and are used for healthy patients receiving routine services, for therapeutic encounters, for a problem that is not currently affecting the patient's condition, and for preoperative evaluations. E codes, which are never used as primary codes, classify the injuries resulting from various environmental events.

5. The three steps in the coding process are to (a) assemble the pertinent documentation, (b) analyze the reason for the encounter that is the patient's primary diagnosis, and (c) assign the code by locating the medical term in the Alphabetic Index and verifying the code in the Tabular List.

6. Three key coding guidelines are (a) code the primary diagnosis first, followed by current coexisting conditions; (b) code to the highest degree of certainty, never coding inconclusive, rule-out diagnoses; and (c) code to the highest level of specificity, using fifth digits or fourth digits when available.

PART 2

Coding Procedures

Objectives

After studying this chapter, you will be able to:

1. Discuss the purpose of CPT.
2. Describe the structure and content of the index and the main text.
3. Interpret the formats, conventions, and symbols used in CPT.
4. Describe the purpose and correct use of modifiers.
5. List the three general steps in the procedural coding process.
6. Discuss the purpose, structure, and key guidelines associated with each of the six sections of CPT codes.
7. Describe the purpose and correct use of HCPCS codes and modifiers.
8. Analyze procedural statements, apply appropriate coding guidelines, and assign correct CPT codes.

Key Terms

add-on code
bundled code
Category II codes
Category III codes
consultation
Current Procedural Terminology (CPT)
descriptor
durable medical equipment (DME)
E/M codes

established patient
fragmented billing
global period
global surgery concept
Healthcare Common Procedure Coding System (HCPCS)
modifier
new patient
outpatient
panel

physical status modifier
primary procedure
professional component
referral
secondary procedure
section guidelines
separate procedure
surgical package
technical component
unbundling
unlisted procedure

Why This Part Is Important to You

Procedure codes, like diagnosis codes, are an important part of the medical billing and reimbursement process. Standard procedure codes are used by physicians in medical practices to report the medical, surgical, and diagnostic services they provide. These codes are used by payers to determine reimbursement levels. Accurate procedural coding ensures that providers receive the maximum appropriate reimbursement for services.

Procedure codes are also used to establish guidelines for the delivery of the best possible care for patients. Researchers track different courses of treatment for patients with similar diagnoses and evaluate patients' outcomes. For example, this type of analysis has shown that patients who have had heart attacks can reduce the risk of subsequent heart attacks by taking a medication called beta blockers.

This part of *Basic Medical Coding* gives you a fundamental understanding of procedural coding principles and guidelines. You also have an opportunity to reinforce this understanding by practicing your coding skills as you complete the Coding Worksheets and take the CPT Coding Quiz.

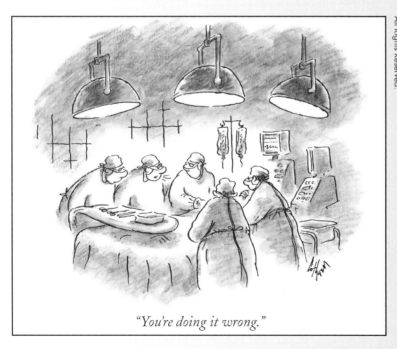

"You're doing it wrong."

CURRENT PROCEDURAL TERMINOLOGY (CPT)

The procedure codes most widely used in the United States are listed in the *Current Procedural Terminology* (referred to as CPT). A publication of the American Medical Association (AMA), CPT contains codes for the procedures and services that are commonly used in medical practices and performed by many physicians across the country.

CPT codes have five digits (with no decimals) followed by a descriptor, which is a brief explanation of the procedure:

99204   Office visit for evaluation and management of a new patient

Although the codes are grouped into sections, such as Surgery, codes from any section can be used by all types of physicians. For example, a family practitioner might use codes from the Surgery section to describe an office procedure such as the incision and drainage of an abscess.

The wide use of CPT codes began in 1983, when the Health Care Financing Administration (now named the Centers for Medicare and Medicaid Services, CMS) standardized codes for physician procedures and services reimbursed by government-sponsored programs, especially Medicare. CMS developed the **Healthcare Common Procedure Coding System** (referred to as **HCPCS** and pronounced hick-picks). From the many different coding systems then in use, CMS chose the AMA's codes as its standard for procedure codes. The current HCPCS is discussed on pages 74–77.

Within a few years after CMS required HCPCS codes for Medicare claims, most insurance companies that were working with both HCPCS and other systems had also adopted CPT codes as their standard. Today, CPT codes are required for submitting electronic health care claims to all payers.

✓ **HIPAA Tip**

Mandated Use of CPT

- CPT is the mandated code set for physician services under HIPAA's Electronic Health Care Transactions and Code Sets.
- CPT procedure codes must be used to bill Medicare and most other payers.

Organization and Format

The manual is made up of the main text—sections of codes—followed by appendixes and an index. The main text has six sections:

- Evaluation and Management   Codes 99201–99499
- Anesthesia   Codes 00100–01999
- Surgery   Codes 10021–69990
- Radiology   Codes 70010–79999
- Pathology and Laboratory   Codes 80048–89356
- Medicine   Codes 90281–99602

Table 2.1 summarizes the types of codes, organization, and guidelines of the six main sections. CPT also contains appendixes and an index, which is provided to make the search for the correct code more efficient.

Updates

Because new procedures and treatments are developed regularly, the AMA publishes a revised CPT each year. The new codes and other changes contained in the annual revision are released by the AMA on

Table 2.1	CPT Sections		
SECTION	**DEFINITION OF CODES**	**STRUCTURE**	**KEY GUIDELINES**
Evaluation and Management	Physicians' services that are performed to determine the best course for patient care	Organized by place and/or type of service	New/established patients; other definitions Unlisted services/special reports Selecting an E/M service level
Anesthesia	Anesthesia services done by or supervised by a physician; includes general, regional, and local anesthesia	Organized by body site	Time-based Services covered (bundled) in codes Unlisted services/special reports Qualifying circumstances codes
Surgery	Surgical procedures performed by physicians	Organized by body system and then body site, followed by procedural groups	Surgical package definition Follow-up care definition Add-on codes Separate procedures Subsection notes Unlisted services/special reports Starred procedures
Radiology	Radiology services done by or supervised by a physician	Organized by type of procedure followed by body site	Unlisted services/special reports Supervision and interpretation (professional and technical components)
Pathology and Laboratory	Pathology and laboratory services done by physicians or by physician-supervised technicians	Organized by type of procedure	Complete procedure Panels Unlisted services/special reports
Medicine	Evaluation, therapeutic, and diagnostic procedures done or supervised by a physician	Organized by type of service or procedure	Subsection notes Multiple procedures reported separately Add-on codes Separate procedures Unlisted services/special reports

October 1 and are in effect for procedures and services provided on or after January 1 of the next year. The CPT annual revision is available in various formats from commercial publishers soon after it is released. Medical specialty societies and the AMA also report the new codes on their Internet Web sites.

HIPAA Tip

Using the Current Codes
Physician practices must be prepared to implement new CPT codes on the date that they become effective. Preparations include updating the codes on encounter forms and billing software. HIPAA requires health care claims to use the procedure codes that are current as of the date of service, so there is no "grace period."

THE INDEX

Like assigning diagnosis codes, selecting a correct procedure code begins by reviewing the physician's statements in the patient's medical record to determine the service, procedure, or treatment that was performed. Then you locate the index entry, which provides a pointer to the correct code range in the main text. Using the CPT index makes the process of selecting procedural codes more efficient. The index contains the descriptive terms that are listed in the sections of codes in the CPT.

Main Terms and Modifying Terms

The main terms in the index are printed in boldface type. There are five types of main terms:

1. The name of the procedure or service, such as echocardiography, extraction, and cast
2. The name of the organ or other anatomical site, such as stomach, wrist, and salivary gland
3. The name of the condition, such as abscess, wound, and postpartum care
4. A synonym or an eponym for the term, such as Noble Procedure, Ramstedt operation, and Fowler-Stephens orchiopexy
5. The abbreviation for the term, such as CAT scan and ECMO

Many terms are listed more than one way. For example, the procedure kidney biopsy is listed both as a procedure—Biopsy, kidney— and by the site—Kidney, biopsy.

A main term may be followed by subterms that further describe the entry. These additional indented terms help in the selection process. For example, the procedure repair of tennis elbow is located beneath *repair* under the main term *elbow* (see Figure 2.1).

Code Ranges

A range of codes is shown when more than one code applies to an entry. Two codes, either sequential or not, are separated by a comma:

Cervix
Biopsy. 57500, 57520

More than two sequential codes are separated by a hyphen:

Dislocation
Ankle
     Closed Treatment 27840-27842

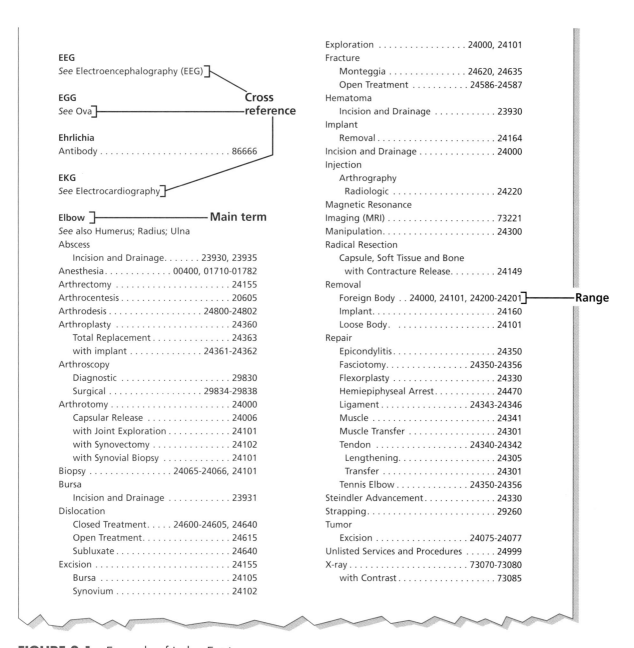

FIGURE 2.1 Example of Index Entries

....

Cross-References and Convention

There are two types of cross-references.

1. *See* is a mandatory instruction. It tells the coder to refer to the term that follows it to find the code. It is used mainly for synonyms, eponyms, and abbreviations. For example, the cross-reference "See Electrocardiography" follows EKG (see Figure 2.1).

2. *See also* tells the coder to look under the term that follows if the procedure is not listed below. For example, under *Elbow*, the cross-reference "See also Humerus; Radius; Ulna" points to those main terms if the entry is not located under *Elbow* (see Figure 2.1).

To save space, some connecting words are left out and must be assumed by the reader. For example:

Ear Cartilage

Graft

      to face. 21235

should be read "graft of ear cartilage to face." The reader supplies the word *of.*

THE MAIN TEXT

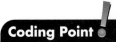

Coding Point

Correct Coding Procedure

Do not select a CPT code only on the basis of the index entry, because often the main text contains additional entries and important guidelines that affect the choice of a correct code.

After you use the index to point to a possible code, read the main text to verify the selection of the code (see Figure 2.2).

Each of the six sections of the main text lists procedure codes and descriptions under subsection headings. These headings group procedures or services, such as Therapeutic or Diagnostic Injections or Psychoanalysis; body systems, such as Digestive System; anatomical sites, such as Abdomen; and tests and examinations, such as Complete Blood Count (CBC). Following these headings are additional subgroups of procedures, systems, or sites. For example, Figure 2.2 shows this structure, in which a body system is the subsection followed by a procedure subgroup:

Surgery Section *<The Section>*

    Musculoskeletal System *<The Subsection>*

        Endoscopy/Arthroscopy *<The Procedure Subgroup>*

The section, subsection, and code number range on a page are shown at the top of the page of the CPT, making it easier to locate a code.

Guidelines

Each section begins with **section guidelines** for the use of its codes. The guidelines cover definitions and items unique to the section. They also include special notes about the structure of the section or the rules for its use. Study the guidelines carefully, and follow them so you can correctly use the codes in the section. Some notes apply only to specific subsections. The guidelines list the subsections that have these notes, and the notes themselves begin that subsection (see Figure 2.2).

Most sections' guidelines give codes for **unlisted procedures**—those not completely described by any code in the CPT. For example, in the Evaluation and Management section, two unlisted codes are provided:

99429   Unlisted preventive medicine service

99499   Unlisted evaluation and management service

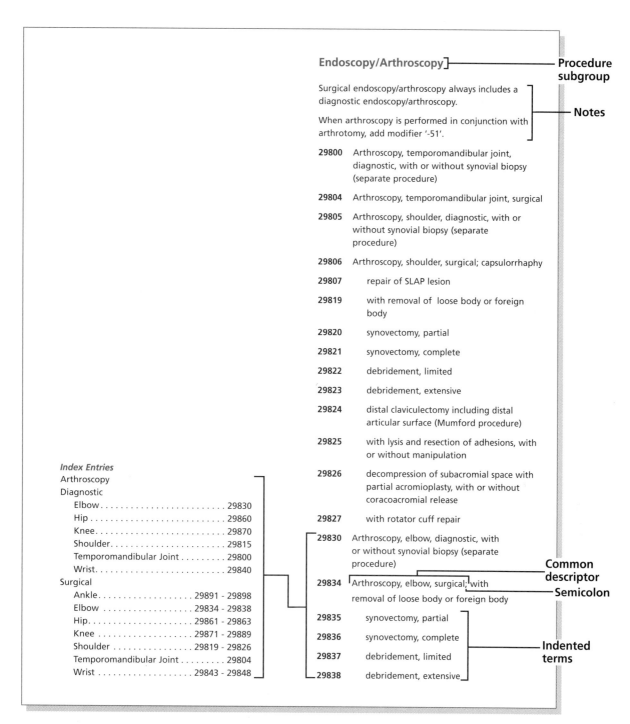

Endoscopy/Arthroscopy — Procedure subgroup

Surgical endoscopy/arthroscopy always includes a diagnostic endoscopy/arthroscopy.

When arthroscopy is performed in conjunction with arthrotomy, add modifier '-51'.

— Notes

29800   Arthroscopy, temporomandibular joint, diagnostic, with or without synovial biopsy (separate procedure)

29804   Arthroscopy, temporomandibular joint, surgical

29805   Arthroscopy, shoulder, diagnostic, with or without synovial biopsy (separate procedure)

29806   Arthroscopy, shoulder, surgical; capsulorrhaphy

29807   repair of SLAP lesion

29819   with removal of loose body or foreign body

29820   synovectomy, partial

29821   synovectomy, complete

29822   debridement, limited

29823   debridement, extensive

29824   distal claviculectomy including distal articular surface (Mumford procedure)

29825   with lysis and resection of adhesions, with or without manipulation

29826   decompression of subacromial space with partial acromioplasty, with or without coracoacromial release

29827   with rotator cuff repair

29830   Arthroscopy, elbow, diagnostic, with or without synovial biopsy (separate procedure)

29834   Arthroscopy, elbow, surgical; with removal of loose body or foreign body
— Common descriptor / Semicolon

29835   synovectomy, partial

29836   synovectomy, complete

29837   debridement, limited

29838   debridement, extensive
— Indented terms

Index Entries
Arthroscopy
Diagnostic
    Elbow 29830
    Hip 29860
    Knee 29870
    Shoulder 29815
    Temporomandibular Joint 29800
    Wrist 29840
Surgical
    Ankle . . . . 29891 - 29898
    Elbow . . . . 29834 - 29838
    Hip . . . . 29861 - 29863
    Knee . . . . 29871 - 29889
    Shoulder . . . . 29819 - 29826
    Temporomandibular Joint 29804
    Wrist . . . . 29843 - 29848

FIGURE 2.2 Example of Code Listings from the Musculoskeletal System Subsection of the Surgery Section

When unlisted codes must be selected, which is rare, a written explanation of the procedure or service is needed. Their use can cause delays in processing claims, and it is better to check with the payer to find out if a temporary code has been created for reporting the service.

Format of CPT Entries

Semicolons and Indentions

To conserve space, CPT uses a semicolon and indentions when a common part of a main entry applies to all the indented entries that follow. For example, in the entries listed below, the procedure partial laryngectomy (hemilaryngectomy) is the common descriptor. It applies to the four unique descriptors after the semicolon— horizontal, laterovertical, anterovertical, and antero-latero-vertical. Note that the common descriptor begins with a capital letter, but the unique descriptors after the semicolon do not.

31370 Partial laryngectomy (hemilaryngectomy); horizontal

31375   laterovertical

31380   anterovertical

31382   antero-latero-vertical

This method shows the relationships among the entries without repeating the common word or words. Follow this example in Figure 2.2:

Example

Index Entry: Arthroscopy, Surgical 29834–29838

Main Text: **29838** Arthroscopy, elbow, surgical; with debridement, extensive

Cross-References

Some codes and descriptors are followed by indented *see* or *use* entries in parentheses, which point to other codes. For example:

82239 Bile acids; total

82240   cholylglycine

(For bile pigments, urine, see 81000–81005)

Examples

Descriptors often contain clarifying examples in parentheses, sometimes with the abbreviation *e.g.* (meaning for example). These provide further descriptions, such as synonyms or examples, but they are not essential to the selection of the code. Here are examples:

87040 Culture, bacterial; blood, with isolation and presumptive identification of isolates (includes anaerobic culture, if appropriate)

50400 Pyeloplasty (Foley Y-pyeloplasty), plastic operation on renal pelvis, with or without plastic operation on ureter, nephropexy, nephrostomy, pyelostomy, or ureteral splinting; simple

50405   complicated (congenital kidney abnormality, secondary pyelosplasty, solitary kidney, calycoplasty)

Symbols for Changed Codes

These symbols have the following meanings when they appear next to CPT codes:

● A bullet (a black circle) indicates a new procedure code. The symbol appears next to the code only the year that it is added.

▲ A triangle indicates that the code's descriptor has changed. It, too, appears in only the year the descriptor is revised.

►◄ Facing triangles (two triangles that face each other) enclose new or revised text other than the code's descriptor.

Symbol for Add-On Codes

A plus sign (+) next to a code in the main text indicates an **add-on code**. Add-on codes describe **secondary procedures** that are commonly carried out in addition to a **primary procedure**. Add-on codes usually use phrases such as *each additional* or *list separately in addition to the primary procedure* to show that they are never used as stand-alone codes. For example, the add-on code +15001 is used after the code for surgical preparation of a free skin graft site (15000) to provide a specific percentage or dimension of body area that was involved beyond the amount covered in the primary procedure.

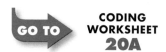

GO TO CODING WORKSHEET **20A**

CATEGORY II AND CATEGORY III CODES

The main codes in CPT are called Category I codes, but in common usage are referred to just as CPT codes. There are two other types of CPT codes, Category II and Category III.

Category II codes are used to track performance measures for a medical goal such as reducing tobacco use. These codes are optional and are not part of reimbursement. They help in the development of best practice care and improve documentation. These codes have an alphabetic character for the fifth digit:

0002F Tobacco use, smoking, assessed

0004F Tobacco use cessation intervention, counseling

Category III codes are temporary codes for emerging technology, services, and procedures. If a Category III code exists for a service, it must be used, rather than an unlisted code. These codes also have an alphabetic character for the fifth digit:

0001T Endovascular repair of infrarenal abdominal aortic aneurysm or dissection

0041T Urinalysis infectious agent detection

A temporary code may become permanent and part of the regular codes if the service it identifies proves effective and is widely performed.

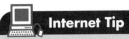

CPT MODIFIERS

A CPT **modifier** is a two-digit number that may be attached to most five-digit procedure codes (see Table 2.2). Modifiers are used to communicate special circumstances involved with a procedure that has been performed. A modifier indicates to private and government payers that the physician considers the procedure to have been altered in some way. A modifier usually affects the normal level of reimbursement for the code to which it is attached.

Table 2.2	CPT Modifiers: Description and Common Use in Main Text Sections						
Code	Description	E/M	Anesthesia	Surgery	Radiology	Pathology	Medicine
-21	Prolonged E/M Service	Yes	Never	Never	Never	Never	Never
-22	Unusual Procedural Service	Never	Yes	Yes	Yes	Yes	Yes
-23	Unusual Anesthesia	Never	Yes				Never
-24	Unrelated E/M Service by the Same Physician During a Postoperative Period	Yes	Never	Never	Never	Never	Never
-25	Significant, Separately Identifiable E/M Service by the Same Physician on the Same Day of the Procedure or Other Service	Yes	Never	Never	Never	Never	Never
-26	Professional Component	—	—	Yes	Yes	Yes	Yes
-32	Mandated Services	Yes	Yes	Yes	Yes	Yes	Yes
-47	Anesthesia by Surgeon	Never	Never	Yes	Never	Never	Never
-50	Bilateral Procedure	—	—	Yes	—	—	—
-51	Multiple Procedures	—	Yes	Yes	Yes	Never	Yes
-52	Reduced Services	Yes	—	Yes	Yes	Yes	Yes
-53	Discontinued Procedure	Never	Yes	Yes	Yes	Yes	Yes
-54	Surgical Care Only	—	—	Yes	—	—	—
-55	Postoperative Management Only	—	—	Yes	—	—	Yes

Table 2.2	CPT Modifiers: Description and Common Use in Main Text Sections, *continued*						
Code	**Description**	**E/M**	**Anesthesia**	**Surgery**	**Radiology**	**Pathology**	**Medicine**
-56	Preoperative Management Only	—	—	Yes	—	—	Yes
-57	Decision for Surgery	Yes	—	—	—	—	Yes
-58	Staged or Related Procedure/Service by the Same Physician During the Postoperative Period	—	—	Yes	Yes	—	Yes
-59	Distinct Procedural Service	—	Yes	Yes	Yes	Yes	Yes
-62	Two Surgeons	Never	Never	Yes	Yes	Never	—
-63	Procedure Performed on Infants	—	—	Yes	Yes	—	Yes
-66	Surgical Team	Never	Never	Yes	Yes	Never	—
-76	Repeat Procedure by Same Physician	—	—	Yes	Yes	—	Yes
-77	Repeat Procedure by Another Physician	—	—	Yes	Yes	—	Yes
-78	Return to the Operating Room for a Related Procedure During the Postoperative Period	—	—	Yes	Yes	—	Yes
-79	Unrelated Procedure/Service by the Same Physician During the Postoperative Period	—	—	Yes	Yes	—	Yes
-80	Assistant Surgeon	Never	—	Yes	Yes	—	—
-81	Minimum Assistant Surgeon	Never	—	Yes	—	—	—
-82	Assistant Surgeon (when qualified resident surgeon not available)	Never	—	Yes	—	—	—
-90	Reference (Outside) Laboratory	—	—	Yes	Yes	Yes	Yes
-91	Repeat Clinical Diagnostic Laboratory Test	—	—	Yes	Yes	Yes	Yes
-99	Multiple Modifiers	—	—	Yes	Yes	—	Yes

Source: CPT 2004

Key:
Yes = commonly used
— = not usually used with the codes in that section
Never = not used with the codes in that section

For example, the modifier -76, Repeat Procedure by Same Physician, is used when the reporting physician repeats a procedure or service after doing the first one. A situation requiring this modifier to show the extra procedure might be:

Procedural Statement: Physician performed a chest X-ray before placing a chest tube and then, after the chest tube was placed, performed a second chest X-ray to verify its position.

Code: **71020-76**   Radiologic examination, chest, two views, frontal and lateral; repeat procedure or service by same physician

The modifiers are listed in Appendix A of CPT. However, not all modifiers are available for use with every section's codes:

- Some modifiers apply only to certain sections. For example, the modifier -21, Prolonged Evaluation and Management Services, is used only with codes that are located in the Evaluation and Management section, as its descriptor implies.

- Add-on codes cannot be modified with -51, Multiple Procedures, because the add-on code is used to add increments to a primary procedure, so the need for multiple procedures is replaced by procedures added on.

- Codes that begin with a circle containing a backslash (Ø) also cannot be modified with -51, "Multiple Procedures."

What Modifiers Mean

The use of a modifier indicates that the procedure was different from the listed descriptor, but not in a way that changed the definition or required a different code. Modifiers are used mainly when

- A procedure has two parts—a **technical component** performed by a technician, such as a radiologist, and a **professional component** that the physician performed, usually the interpretation and reporting of the results
- A service or procedure was performed more than once, by more than one physician, and/or in more than one location
- A service or procedure has been increased or reduced
- Only part of a procedure was done
- A bilateral or multiple procedure was performed
- Unusual difficulties occurred during the procedure

Assigning Modifiers

Modifiers are shown by adding a hyphen and the two-digit code to the CPT code. For example, a physician providing therapeutic radiology services in a hospital would report the modifier -26, Professional Component, as follows:

73090-26

This format means professional component only for an X-ray of the forearm. (In effect, it means that the physician who performed the service did not own the equipment used, so the fee is "split" between the physician and the equipment owner.)

Two or more modifiers may be used with one code to give the most accurate description possible. The use of two or more modifiers is shown by reporting -99, Multiple Modifiers, followed by the other modifiers listed with the most essential modifier first.

Procedures: Multitrauma patient's extremely difficult surgery after a car accident; team surgery by orthopedic surgeon and neurosurgeon. The first surgical procedure carries these modifiers:

27236-99, -66, -51, -22

Some procedures have a pair of codes, one for a unilateral service and another for a bilateral service. Others are bilateral, applying to both anatomical parts or sections. For example, the audiologic function test codes describe tests on both ears. In other cases, codes are unilateral and require a -50 modifier when performed on both parts or sections.

If a procedure with a bilateral code is performed on just one of the two parts, a modifier is also needed. Use the -52 modifier, reduced services, to show that half the work described by the code was done.

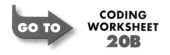

GO TO

CODING WORKSHEET 20B

THE APPENDIXES

The five appendixes contain information helpful to the coding process:

1. *Appendix A—Modifiers:* A complete listing of all modifiers with descriptions and, in some cases, examples of usage
2. *Appendix B—Summary of Additions, Deletions, and Revisions:* A summary of the codes added, revised, and deleted in the current version
3. *Appendix C—Clinical Examples:* Case examples of the proper use of the codes in the Evaluation and Management section
4. *Appendix D—Summary of Add-on Codes:* List of supplemental codes used for procedures that are commonly done in addition to the primary procedure
5. *Appendix E—Summary of Codes Exempt from Modifier -51:* Codes to which the modifier showing multiple procedures cannot be attached because they already include a multiple descriptor

✓ **HIPAA Tip**

CPT ASSISTANT

The American Medical Association's monthly publication *CPT Assistant* is the authoritative guide to the correct use of CPT codes.

CODING STEPS

The process for assigning correct procedure codes has three steps. This process applies to the six sections of CPT, as will be discussed in the following sections.

Step 1 Analyze the Procedures and Services to Report

The first step is to review the documentation of the patient's visit and decide which procedures and/or services were performed. Then, based on knowledge of the CPT and of the payer's policies, a decision is made about which services can be charged and are to be coded to report on health care claims.

Step 2 Assign the Correct Codes

Follow this process to select a code:

1. Use the index to locate the main term for each procedure or service. If the term is not found, look up the organ or body site, and then the disease or injury. Further checking can be done to locate any synonyms, eponyms, or abbreviations associated with the main term. Review the entries under the main term to see if any apply, and check cross-references.

2. If you cannot locate the main term in the index, review the main term with the physician for clarification. In some cases, there is an alternative term that can be used.

3. Review the main text listing, including all section guidelines and notes for the particular subsection, to make the final code choice. Services that cannot be billed separately because they are covered under another, broader code are eliminated.

4. Rank the codes to be reported for each day's services in order of highest to lowest rate of reimbursement. The actual order in which they were performed on a particular day is not important. When reporting, the earliest date of service is listed first, followed by subsequent dates of service. For example:

Date	Procedure	Charge
11/17/2006	**99204**	$202
11/20/2006	**43215**	$355
11/20/2006	**74235**	$75

Step 3 Analyze the Need for Modifiers

The circumstances involved with the procedure or service may require the use of modifiers. The patient's diagnosis may affect this determination. Appropriate modifiers are appended to the procedure codes.

EVALUATION AND MANAGEMENT CODES

The codes in the Evaluation and Management section (E/M codes) cover physicians' services that are performed to determine the best course for patient care. The E/M codes are listed first in CPT because they are used so frequently by all types of physicians. Often called the cognitive codes, the E/M codes cover the complex process physicians use to gather and analyze information about a patient's illness and make decisions about the patient's condition and the best treatment or course of management. The actual treatments—such as surgical procedures and injections—are covered in the CPT sections that follow the E/M codes, such as the Anesthesia and Surgery sections.

Patients' conditions require different levels of information gathering, analysis, and decision making by physicians. For example, on the low end of a range might be a patient with a mild case of poison ivy. On the opposite end is a patient with a life-threatening condition. The E/M codes reflect these different levels. There are five codes for an office visit with a new patient, for example, and another five for office visits with established patients. A financial value (fee or prospective payment) is assigned by payers to each code in a range. To justify the use of a higher-level code in the range—one that is tied to a higher value—physicians must perform and document specific clinical facts about patient encounters.

Structure

Most codes in the E/M section are organized by the place of service. A few (for example, consultations) are grouped by type of service. The subsections are as follows:

Office or Other Outpatient Services

Hospital Observation Services

Hospital Inpatient Services

Consultations

Emergency Department Services

Pediatric Critical Care Patient Transport

Critical Care Services

Neonatal and Pediatric Critical Care Services

Pediatric Critical Care

Neonatal Critical Care

Intensive (Non-Critical) Low Birth Weight Service

Nursing Facility Services

Domiciliary, Rest Home, or Custodial Care Services

Home Services

Prolonged Services

Case Management Services

Care Plan Oversight Services

Preventive Medicine Services

Newborn Care

Special/Other E/M Services

A New or an Established Patient?

Many subsections of E/M codes assign different code ranges for new patients and established patients. A **new patient** has not received any professional services from the physician (or from another physician of the same specialty in the same group practice) within the past three years. An **established patient** has received professional services under those conditions. The distinction is important because new patients typically require more effort by the physician and practice staff and should therefore be rated at a higher value.

The term *any professional services* in the definitions of new and established patients means that if a patient had a face-to-face encounter with a physician, the established category is used. The same rule applies to a patient of a physician who moves to another group practice. If the patient then sees the physician (or another of the same specialty) in the new practice, the patient is established. In other words, the patient is new to the practice, but established to the provider. Figure 2.3 presents a decision tree for determining the patient's status.

A Consultation or a Referral?

To understand the subsection of E/M codes on consultations requires a review of the difference between a consultation and a referral in coding terminology. A **consultation** occurs when a second physician, at the request of the patient's physician (the attending or treating physician), examines the patient. The second physician usually focuses on a particular issue and reports a written opinion to the first physician. The physician providing a

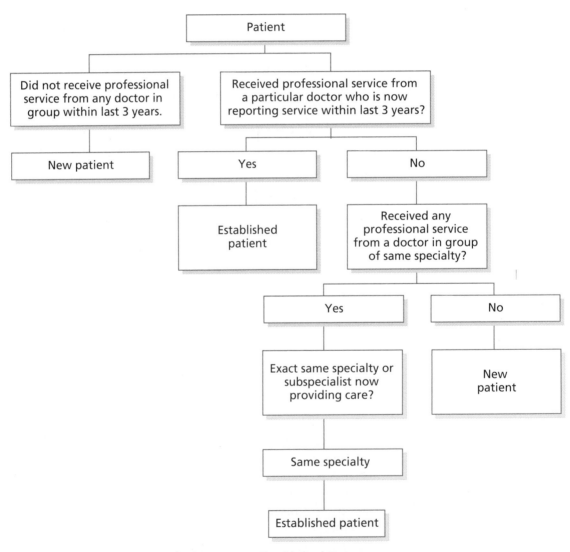

FIGURE 2.3 Decision Tree for New versus Established Patients

consultation may perform a service for the patient, but does not independently start a full course of treatment (although the consulting physician may recommend one) or take charge of the patient's care. Consultations require use of the E/M consultation codes (the range from 99241 to 99275).

On the other hand, when the patient is given a referral, either the total care or a specific portion of care is transferred to another physician. The patient becomes a new patient of that doctor and may not return to the care of the referring physician until the completion of a course of treatment. Referrals require use of the regular office visit E/M service codes.

E/M Modifiers

These modifiers are commonly used to indicate special circumstances involved with evaluation and management services:

-21 *Prolonged Evaluation and Management service:* Used when the services are greater than the highest level described for the code range.

-24 *Unrelated Evaluation and Management service by the same physician during a postoperative period:* Used when an E/M service that is not related to the reason for the surgery is provided within the postoperative time period included in the payer's reimbursement.

-25 *Significant, separately identifiable Evaluation and Management service by the same physician on the same day of the procedure or other service:* Used when the physician provides an E/M service in addition to another E/M service or a procedure on the same day. The E/M service to which the modifier is appended must be significant enough to report.

-32 *Mandated services:* Used when the procedure is required by a payer.

-52 *Reduced services:* Used when an E/M service is less extensive than the descriptor indicates.

-57 *Decision for surgery:* Used to indicate the visit where the decision for surgery was made and the patient was counseled about risks and outcomes.

E/M Code Selection

To select the correct E/M code, follow eight steps (see Figure 2.4 on page 52), as explained below.

Step 1 Determine the Category and Subcategory of Service Based on the Location of Service and the Patient's Status

Use the list of E/M categories, such as office visits, hospital services, and preventive medicine services, to locate the appropriate place or type of service in the index. In the main text of the selected category, then choose the subcategory, such as new or established patient.

Documentation: initial hospital visit for established patient

Index: Hospital Services

> Inpatient Services

> > Initial Care, New or Established Patient

Code Ranges: 99221–99223

STEP 1   Determine the category and subcategory of service based on the location of service and the patient's status

STEP 2   Determine the extent of the history that is documented

STEP 3   Determine the extent of the examination that is documented

STEP 4   Determine the complexity of medical decision making that is documented

STEP 5   Analyze the requirements to report the service level

STEP 6   Verify the service level based on the nature of the presenting problem, time, counseling, and care coordination

STEP 7   Verify that the documentation is complete

STEP 8   Assign the code

FIGURE 2.4   Selecting an Evaluation and Management Code

For most types of service, such as initial hospital care for an established patient, between three and five codes are listed. To select an appropriate code from this range, consider three key components: (1) the history the physician documented, (2) the examination that was documented, and (3) the medical decisions the physician documented. (The exception to this guideline is selecting a code for counseling or coordination of care, where the amount of time the physician spends may be the only key component.)

Step 2   Determine the Extent of the History That Is Documented

History is the information the physician received by questioning the patient about the chief complaint and other signs or symptoms, about all or selected body systems, and about pertinent past history, family background, and other personal factors. If the patient is incapacitated, the history may be taken from a family member.

The history is documented in the patient medical record as follows:

- *History of present illness (HPI):* The history of the illness is a description of the development of the illness from the first sign or symptom that the patient experienced to the present time. It includes everything related to the illness or condition, such as the severity, location, and timing of pain, and other signs and symptoms.

- *Review of systems (ROS):* The review of systems is an inventory of body systems. These systems are constitutional symptoms (such as fever or weight loss); eyes; ears, nose, mouth, and throat;

cardiovascular (CV); respiratory; gastrointestinal (GI); genitourinary (GU); musculoskeletal; integumentary; neurological; psychiatric; endocrine; hematologic/lymphatic; and allergic/immunologic.

- *Past medical history (PMH):* The past history of the patient's experiences with illnesses, injuries, and treatments contains data about other major illnesses and injuries, operations, and hospitalizations. It also covers current medications the patient is taking, allergies, immunization status, and diet.

- *Family history (FH):* The family history reviews the medical events in the patient's family. It includes the health status or cause of death of parents, brothers and sisters, and children; specific diseases that are related to the patient's chief complaint or the patient's diagnosis; and the presence of any known hereditary diseases.

- *Social history (SH):* The facts gathered in the social history, which depend on the patient's age, include marital status, employment, and other factors.

The histories documented after the HPI are sometimes referred to as PFSH, for past, family, and social history.

The history that the physician obtains is categorized by the coder as one of four types:

1. *Problem-focused:* Determining the patient's chief complaint and obtaining a brief history of the present illness

2. *Expanded problem-focused:* Determining the patient's chief complaint and obtaining a brief history of the present illness, plus a problem-pertinent system review of the particular body system that is involved

3. *Detailed:* Determining the chief complaint; obtaining an extended history of the present illness; reviewing both the problem-pertinent system and additional systems; and taking pertinent past, family, and/or social history

4. *Comprehensive:* Determining the chief complaint and taking an extended history of the present illness, a complete review of systems, and a complete past, family, and social history

EXTENT OF HISTORY	History of Present Illness (HPI)	Review of Systems (ROS)	Past/Family/Social History (PFSH)
PROBLEM-FOCUSED	Brief	None	None
EXPANDED PROBLEM-FOCUSED	Brief	Problem-Pertinent	None
DETAILED	Extended	Extended	Problem-Pertinent
COMPREHENSIVE	Extended	Complete	Complete

Step 3 Determine the Extent of the Examination That Is Documented

The physician may examine a particular body area or organ system or may conduct a multisystem examination. The body areas are divided into the head and face; chest, including breasts and axilla; abdomen; genitalia, groin, and buttocks; back; and each extremity. The organ systems that may be examined are the eyes; the ears, nose, mouth, and throat; cardiovascular; respiratory; gastrointestinal; genitourinary; musculoskeletal; skin; neurologic; psychiatric; and hematologic/lymphatic/immunologic.

The examination that the physician performs is assigned by the coder into one of these types:

1. *Problem-focused:* A limited examination of the affected body area or system

2. *Expanded problem-focused:* A limited examination of the affected body area or system and other related areas

3. *Detailed:* An extended examination of the affected body area or system and other related areas

4. *Comprehensive:* A general multisystem examination or a complete examination of a single organ system

The coder analyzes the documentation of the examination to decide which type has been done.

Step 4 Determine the Complexity of Medical Decision Making That Is Documented

The complexity of the medical decisions that the physician makes involves how many possible diagnoses or treatment options were considered; how much information (such as test results or previous records) was considered in analyzing the patient's problem; and how serious the illness is, meaning how much risk there is for significant complications, advanced illness, or death.

Coding Point

Documentation Guidelines

Two sets of guidelines for deciding on the level of the exam have been published by CMS and the AMA, the 1995 Documentation Guidelines for Evaluation and Management Services and a 1997 version. CMS permits providers to use either the 1995 or the 1997 E/M guidelines. The guidelines are similar; the 1997 version has a more detailed counting method for the exam. As a practical matter, the coder needs to know which guidelines are in use for the services being coded.

The decisions that the physician makes are categorized by the coder as one of four types:

1. *Straightforward:* Minimal diagnoses options, a minimal amount of data, and minimum risk
2. *Low complexity:* Limited diagnoses options, a low amount of data, and low risk
3. *Moderate complexity:* Multiple diagnoses options, a moderate amount of data, and moderate risk
4. *High complexity:* Extensive diagnoses options, an extensive amount of data, and high risk

COMPLEXITY OF MEDICAL DECISION MAKING	Diagnoses Options	Data Reviewed	Risks
STRAIGHTFORWARD	Few	Little or none	Minimal
LOW COMPLEXITY	Limited	Limited	Low
MODERATE COMPLEXITY	Many	Moderate	Moderate
HIGH COMPLEXITY	Extensive	Extensive	High

Step 5 Analyze the Requirements to Report the Service Level

The descriptor for each E/M code explains the standards for its use. For office visits and most other services to new patients, and for initial care visits, all three of the key component requirements must be met. For example, to choose code 99203, CPT states that a detailed history, detailed examination, and low-level decision making must be documented. This is printed in CPT as follows:

99203 **Office or other outpatient visit** for the evaluation and management of a new patient, which require these three key components:

- **a detailed history**
- **a detailed examination**
- **medical decision making of low complexity**

For most services for established patients and for subsequent care visits, two out of three of the key component requirements must be met. For example, to select code 99232, CPT states:

99232 **Subsequent hospital care**, per day, for the evaluation and management of a patient, which requires at least two of these three key components:

- **an expanded problem-focused interval history**
- **an expanded problem-focused examination**
- **medical decision making of moderate complexity**

Step 6 Verify the Service Level Based on the Nature of the Presenting Problem, Time, Counseling, and Care Coordination

Many E/M code descriptors mention two additional components: (1) how severe the patient's condition is, referred to as the nature of the presenting problem, and (2) how much time the physician typically spends directly treating the patient. These factors, while not the key components, are used by the coder to verify that the correct service level is selected. For example, this statement appears after the 99214 code (office visit for the evaluation and management of an established patient):

Usually, the presenting problem(s) are of moderate to high severity. Physicians typically spend 25 minutes face-to-face with the patient and/or family.

Counseling is a discussion with a patient regarding areas such as diagnostic results, instructions for follow-up treatment, and patient education. It is mentioned as a typical part of each E/M service in the descriptor, but it is not required to be documented as a key component. Coordination of care with other providers or agencies is also mentioned. When coordination of care is provided but the patient is not present, codes from the case management and care plan oversight services subsections are reported.

Step 7 Verify That the Documentation Is Complete

Meeting the requirements means that the documentation must contain the record of the physician's work. When an E/M code is assigned, the patient's medical record must contain the clinical details to support it. The history, examination, and medical decision making must be sufficiently documented so that the medical necessity and appropriateness of the service can be understood.

Step 8 Assign the Code and Modifiers, If Appropriate

The code that has been selected is assigned. The need for any modifiers, based on the documentation of special circumstances, is also reviewed.

Reporting E/M Codes: Other Considerations

Office versus Hospital Services

Office and other outpatient services are the most often reported E/M services. A patient is an **outpatient** unless admitted to a health care facility, such as a hospital or nursing home, for a twenty-four-hour period or longer.

- When a patient is evaluated and then admitted to a health care facility, the service is reported using the codes for initial hospital care (the range 99221–99223).
- The admitting physician uses the initial hospital care services codes. Only one provider can report these services; other physicians involved in the patient's care, such as a surgeon or radiologist, use other E/M service codes or other codes from appropriate sections.

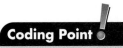

Coding Point

"Initial" E/M Codes

Codes for initial observation care, initial hospital care, and initial inpatient consultation should be reported by a physician only once for a patient admission.

Confirmatory Consultations

Consultations requested by the patient or family members, not the attending physician, are called confirmatory consultations, and are reported using codes 99271 to 99275.

Emergency Department Services

An emergency department is one that is hospital-based and available to patients 24 hours a day. When the physician work in emergency departments is coded, whether the patient is new or established is not applicable. Time is not a factor in selecting the E/M service code. The code ranges are 99281 to 99288.

Preventive Medicine Services

Preventive medicine services are used to report routine physical examinations in the absence of a patient complaint. These codes, in the range 99381 to 99429, are divided according to the age of the patient. Immunizations and other services, such as lab tests that are normal parts of an annual physical, are reported using the appropriate codes from the Medicine and the Pathology and Laboratory sections (see pages 71 and 72).

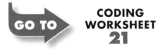

GO TO   **CODING WORKSHEET 21**

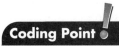

Coding Point

Modifier -25

During a routine physical examination, an illness or clinical sign of a condition may be found that requires the physician to conduct an additional evaluation. In this case, the preventive medicine service code is reported first, followed by the appropriate E/M code for the new problem, adding the -25 modifier, Significant, Separate E/M Service.

ANESTHESIA CODES

The codes in the Anesthesia section are used for anesthesia services performed or supervised by a physician. These services include general and regional anesthesia, as well as supplementation of local anesthesia. The main anesthesia codes are bundled codes, under which a group of related procedures are covered by a single code. These bundled codes include the usual services of an anesthesiologist:

- Usual preoperative visits for evaluation and planning
- Care during the procedure, such as administering fluid or blood, placing monitoring devices or IV lines, laryngoscopy, interpreting lab data, and nerve stimulation
- Routine postoperative care

Example

Anesthesiologist Report: Initial meeting with seven-year-old patient in good health, determined good candidate for required general anesthesia for tonsillectomy. Surgical procedure conducted April 4, 2006; patient in the supine position; administered general anesthesia via endotracheal tube. Routine monitoring during procedure. Following successful removal of the right and left tonsils, the patient was awakened and taken to the recovery room in satisfactory condition.

00170-P1   Anesthesia for intraoral procedures, including biopsy; not otherwise specified

(The modifier -P1 is discussed below.)

Postoperative critical care and pain management requested by the surgeon are not routine and are not included in a bundled code. Such additional procedures done by an anesthesiologist can be reported.

Anesthesia codes are reimbursed according to time. The American Society of Anesthesiologists assigns a base unit value to each code. The anesthesiologist also records the amount of time spent with the patient during the procedure and adds this to the base value. Difficulties, such as a patient with severe systemic disease, also add to the value of the anesthesiologist's services.

Coding Point

Unbundling

Unbundling occurs when separate procedures are reported that should have been included under a bundled code. This billing practice is not legal and will result in claim denial.

Structure

The Anesthesia section's subsections are organized by body site. Under each subsection, the codes are arranged by procedures. For example, under the heading *Neck*, codes for procedures performed on various parts of the neck (the integumentary system; the esophagus, thyroid, larynx, trachea; and lymphatic system; and the major vessels) are listed. The body-site subsections are followed by two subsections: (1) radiological procedures—that is, anesthesia services for patients receiving diagnostic or therapeutic radiology—and (2) other or unlisted procedures.

Modifiers

Two types of modifiers are used with anesthesia codes: (1) a modifier that describes the patient's physical status and (2) the standard CPT modifiers.

Physical Status Modifiers

Because the patient's health has a large effect on the level of difficulty of anesthesia services, anesthesia codes must be assigned a **physical status modifier**. This modifier is added to the code. The patient's physical status is selected from this list:

P1   Normal, healthy patient

P2   Patient with mild systemic disease

P3   Patient with severe systemic disease

P4   Patient with severe systemic disease that is a constant threat to life

P5   Moribund patient who is not expected to survive without the operation

P6   Declared brain-dead patient whose organs are being removed for donation purposes

For example:

00320-P3   Anesthesia services provided to patient with severe diabetes for procedure on larynx

Standard CPT Anesthesia Modifiers

These standard modifiers are also commonly used with anesthesia codes:

-22   *Unusual procedural service:* Used with rare, unusual, or variable anesthesia services.

-23   *Unusual anesthesia service:* Used when the procedure normally requires either no anesthesia or local anesthesia but, because of usual circumstances, general anesthesia is administered.

-32   *Mandated service:* Used when the procedure is required by a payer. For example, a PPO may require an independent evaluation of a patient before procedures are performed.

-51   *Multiple procedures:* Used to identify a second procedure or multiple procedures during the same operation.

-53   *Discontinued:* Used when the procedure is canceled after induction of anesthesia but before the incision is made. If the surgery is canceled after the evaluation of the patient, an E/M code is used rather than this modifier.

-59   *Distinct procedural service:* Used for a different encounter or procedure for the same patient on the same day; also used to describe the requirement for critical care and nonroutine pain management.

Note that modifier -37, Anesthesia by Surgeon, is used only during surgical procedures, not for services performed by anesthesiologists or anesthetists or supervised by surgeons.

For example, an anesthesia code with both types of modifiers appears as:

00320-P3-53   Anesthesia services provided to patient with severe diabetes for procedure on larynx; procedure discontinued because patient experienced a sudden drop in blood pressure

Add-On Codes for Qualifying Circumstances

Four add-on codes are used to indicate that the administration of the anesthesia involved important circumstances that had an effect on how it was performed. As add-on codes, these do not stand alone, but always appear in addition to the primary procedure code. These four codes apply only to anesthesia and are described in the notes for the Anesthesia Section.

+99100   Anesthesia for patient of extreme age (under one year or over age 70)

+99116   Anesthesia complicated by utilization of total body hypothermia

+99135   Anesthesia complicated by utilization of controlled hypotension

+99140   Anesthesia complicated by specified emergency conditions

Assigning Anesthesia Codes

Anesthesia services for Medicare patients and most other patients are reported using codes from the Anesthesia section. However, be aware that some private payers require anesthesia services to be reported by procedure codes from the Surgery section rather than by codes from the Anesthesia section. The anesthesia modifier is added to the procedure code.

GO TO
CODING WORKSHEET 22

> ✓ **HIPAA Tip**
>
> **HCPCS Anesthesia Modifiers**
> Medicare uses additional modifiers for anesthesia services. Part of the HCPCS codes (see Table 2.4 on pages 76–77), these modifiers help clarify special situations when Medicare patient services are reported.

SURGERY CODES

The codes in the Surgery section are used for the many hundreds of surgical procedures performed by physicians. This is the largest procedure code section, with codes ranging from 10021 to 69990. It has these subsections:

Integumentary System   Male Genital System

Musculoskeletal System   Intersex Surgery

Respiratory System   Female Genital System

Cardiovascular System   Maternity Care and Delivery

Hemic and Lymphatic Systems   Endocrine System

Mediastinum and Diaphragm   Nervous System

Digestive System   Eye and Ocular Adnexa

Urinary System   Operating Microscope

The Surgery Section Guidelines contain both general information and a listing of the subsections that have unique special instructions. Read these notes carefully before selecting codes from the procedures that follow them.

Organization of Surgery Codes

Most of the major system subsections are organized anatomically, covering body parts from head to toe. Within this organization, codes are listed in groups of related types of procedures. For example:

Subsection:	DIGESTIVE SYSTEM
Site:	Lips
Heading—type of procedure:	Excision
Description—specific procedure:	**40490** Biopsy of lip

Typical groupings of procedures are

- Incisions: procedures that involve cutting into, such as those with the ending -otomy or -tomy (for example, tracheotomy)

- Excisions: procedures that involve surgical removal, such as those with the ending -ectomy (for example, lumpectomy). Other terms are biopsy, resection, or removal; radical resection means total excision.

- Introduction or removal, amputation

- Repair/revision/reconstruction (-orrhaphy, -oplasty)

- Manipulation or reduction

- Fixation or fusion (-opexy)

- Endoscopic or laparoscopic procedures

Note that many surgical procedures can be performed in more than one way or via more than one approach. Open surgical procedures are performed by creating a surgical incision to access the site. For some of these, the alternative use of the endoscope permits a less-invasive procedure. Endoscopic procedures frequently listed in the Surgery Section include laparoscopy, colonoscopy, bronchoscopy, esophagoscopy, and arthroscopy. These procedures are performed using endoscopic equipment. For example, a laparoscope is an endoscope designed to examine the contents of the peritoneum through a small incision. An arthroscope is an endoscope designed to view the interior of a joint. These are diagnostic endoscopic procedures; the instruments are also used for surgical procedures. Other open procedures may be endoscopically assisted. Coders study the terminology used to identify the technique that has been used.

Surgical Package

Most surgical codes are bundled codes. They include:

- After the decision for surgery, one related E/M encounter on the date immediately before or on the date of the procedure
- The operation: preparing the patient for surgery, including injection of local/topical anesthesia (by the surgeon), and performing the operation, including normal additional procedures, such as debridement
- Typical postoperative follow-up care

The following case shows how the procedural elements—the operation, the use of a local anesthetic, and postoperative care—are covered under a single code.

Example

Procedural Statement: Procedure conducted two weeks ago in office to correct hallux valgus (bunions) on both feet; local nerve block administered, correction by simple exostectomy. Saw patient in office today for routine follow-up; complete healing.

Code: **28290-50**   Bunion correction on both feet

In the Surgery section, the grouping of related activities under a single procedure code is called a surgical package or global surgery concept. Payers assign a fee to a surgical package code that reimburses all the services provided under it. The period of time that is covered for pre-procedure and follow-up care is referred to as the global period. For example, the global period for flexor tendon repair may be set at 0/15, which means no days before the procedure and fifteen days post-procedure. After the global period ends, additional services that are provided can be reported separately for additional payment.

Surgical package codes are assigned single fees. Reporting as a separate procedure anything that is included in the surgical package code is considered unbundling, or fragmented billing. This practice, as noted earlier, causes denied claims and may result in an audit.

Two types of services are not included in surgical package codes. These services are reported separately and reimbursed in addition to the surgical package fee.

- Complications or recurrences that arise after therapeutic surgical procedures.
- Care for the condition for which a diagnostic surgical procedure is performed. Routine follow-up care included in the code refers only to care related to recovery from the diagnostic procedure itself, not the condition. For example, a diagnostic colonoscopy may be performed to examine a growth in the patient's colon. An office visit

after the surgery to evaluate the patient for chemotherapy because the tumor is cancerous is billed separately, not with code 99024 for a postoperative follow-up visit included in the global service.

Separate Procedures

Some procedural code descriptors in the Surgery section are followed by the words *separate procedure* in parentheses. **Separate procedure** means that the procedure is usually done as an integral part of a surgical package—usually a larger procedure—but in some situations, it is not. If a separate procedure is performed alone or along with other procedures but for a separate purpose, it may be reported separately. For example:

42870   Excision or destruction lingual tonsil, any method (separate procedure)

Lingual tonsil excision is a separate procedure. It is usually a part of a routine tonsillectomy, and so cannot be reported separately when a tonsillectomy is performed. When it is done independently, however, this code can be reported.

Radiological Supervision and Interpretation

Often the physician supervises and interprets radiological imaging such as X rays in the course of performing surgery. When the physician provides radiological supervision and interpretation (S&I), a professional component modifier (-26) is attached to the radiology code that is reported with the surgery codes.

The appropriate radiology code or code range is mentioned with the associated surgery codes in CPT. If more than one code is mentioned, the coder turns to the Radiology Section and examines the listed codes to select the correct option. In some cases, separate codes are listed for the professional and the technical components of the service.

Note that the professional component modifier is not used if the physician owns the equipment, provides the supplies, and employs the technicians used for the radiological imaging. In that case, the physician is providing the complete service, and the modifier is not appropriate.

Surgery Modifiers

These modifiers are commonly used to indicate special circumstances involved with surgical procedures:

-22   *Unusual procedural service:* Used with rare, unusual, or variable surgery services; requires documentation.

-26   *Professional component:* Used to report the professional components when a procedure has both professional and technical components.

-32   *Mandated service:* Used when the procedure is required by a payer or governmental, legislative, or regulatory requirement.

-47   *Anesthesia by surgeon:* Used when the surgeon (rather than an anesthesiologist) administers regional or general anesthesia (local/topical anesthesia is bundled in the surgical code).

-50 *Bilateral procedure:* Used to indicate that identical bilateral procedures were performed during the same operation, either through the same incision or on separate body parts, such as left and right bunion correction. Under the guidelines, attaching the bilateral modifier to the code for the first procedure indicates that the procedure was done bilaterally. For example, to report a puncture aspiration of one cyst in each breast:

19100-<u>50</u> Puncture aspiration of cyst of breast

-51 *Multiple procedures:* Used to identify a second procedure or multiple procedures during the same operation. The additional procedures are the same type and done to the same body system. The modifier is attached to the second procedure code. For example, to report two procedures, a bunionectomy on the great toe and, in the same session, correction of a hammertoe on the fourth toe:

28290 Hallux valgus (bunions) correction

28285-<u>51</u> Hammertoe operation, one

-52 *Reduced services:* Used to indicate a procedure that is less extensive than described. The modifier is attached to the procedure code. It is not used to identify a reduced or a discounted fee. Instead, usually, the normal fee is listed, and the payer determines the amount of the reduction.

-53 *Discontinued procedure:* Used when the procedure is discontinued due to circumstances that threaten the patient's well-being—for example, surgery discontinued because the patient went into shock during the operation.

-54 *Surgical care only:* Added to the surgery code when the surgeon performs only the surgery itself, without preoperative or postoperative services. The fee is reduced to reflect only that part of the surgical package.

-55 *Postoperative management only:* Added to the surgery code when the physician provides only the follow-up care in the global period after another physician has done the surgery. The fee is reduced to reflect only that part of the surgical package.

-56 *Preoperative management only:* Added to the surgery code when the physician provides only preoperative care. The fee is reduced to reflect only that part of the surgical package.

-58 *Staged or related procedure or service by the same physician during the postoperative period:* Used when the physician performs a post-operative procedure (1) as planned during the surgery to be done later, (2) that is more extensive than the original procedure, or (3) for therapy after diagnostic surgery.

-59 *Distinct procedural service:* Used for a different encounter or procedure for the same patient on the same day. Either a different patient encounter, an unrelated procedure, a different body site or system, or a separate incision or injury must be involved. It may also be used to describe the requirement for critical care and non-routine pain management. If a separate procedure is performed with other procedures, the modifier -59 is added to the separate code to show that it is a distinct, independent procedure, not part of a surgical package.

-62 *Two surgeons:* Used when a specific surgical procedure requires two surgeons, usually of different specialties; each appends the modifier to the surgical code. Usually each surgeon performs a distinct part of the procedure and dictates a separate operative report. If each surgeon reports different surgical procedure codes, the modifier is not used.

-63 *Procedure performed on infants:* Used when the patient is under twenty-four months of age.

-66 *Surgical team:* Used in very complex procedures that usually require the simultaneous services of physicians of different specialties. Usually used only to report transplant-type procedures.

-76 *Repeat procedure by same physician:* Used when a physician repeats a procedure performed earlier.

-77 *Repeat procedure by another physician:* Used when a physician repeats a procedure done by another physician.

-78 *Return to the operating room for a related procedure during the post-operative period:* Used when the patient develops a complication during the postoperative period that requires an additional procedure by the same physician.

-79 *Unrelated procedure or service by the same physician during the postoperative period:* Used when a second, unrelated surgical procedure is performed by the same physician during the postoperative period.

-80 *Assistant surgeon:* Used when a physician assists another during a surgical procedure. Each physician reports the services using the same code, but the assistant surgeon appends the modifier to the code.

-81 *Minimum assistant surgeon:* Used when an assistant surgeon assists another during only part of a surgical procedure.

-82 *Assistant surgeon (when qualified resident surgeon not available):* Used in teaching hospitals where residents usually assist with surgery but none was available during the reported procedure, so a surgeon performed the assistant's work.

-90 *Reference (outside) laboratory:* Used when laboratory procedures are done by someone other than the reporting physician.

-91 *Repeat clinical diagnostic laboratory test:* Used when laboratory procedures are repeated.

-99 *Multiple modifiers:* Used when more than one modifier is required; the -99 modifier is appended to the basic procedure, followed by the other modifiers in descending order.

Surgery: Integumentary System— Codes 10040–19499

GO TO CODING WORKSHEET 23

The codes in this subsection of CPT's Surgery section cover procedures performed on the integumentary system. Procedures on the skin, subcutaneous and accessory structures, nails, and breast are described. Integumentary system services also include wound and burn repairs as well as skin grafts.

The guidelines for many groupings of procedures, such as paring, excision, or destruction, indicate which specific services are included. For example, shaving of lesions includes local aesthesia and chemical or electrocauterization of the wound. Such services cannot be reported in addition to the code for the procedure.

Surgery: Musculoskeletal System— Codes 20000–29909

GO TO CODING WORKSHEET 24

The codes in this subsection of CPT's Surgery section cover procedures performed on the musculoskeletal system. General procedures, such as wound treatments, excision services, and grafts, are listed first. Codes are then grouped by body site, beginning with the head and ending with the foot. Each body site has the same organization: incision, excision, introduction/removal, repair/revision/reconstruction, fracture/dislocation, manipulation, arthrodesis (fusion or fixation), amputation, and other procedures. Casts/strapping and endoscopy/arthroscopy are the final code groups in the subsection.

Surgery: Respiratory System— Codes 30000–32999

GO TO CODING WORKSHEET 25

The codes in this surgical subsection of CPT cover procedures performed on the respiratory system. Codes are grouped by body site: the nose, accessory sinuses, larynx, trachea and bronchi, and lungs and pleura. Each body site is organized by the type of procedure as appropriate: incision, excision, repair, introduction, and endoscopic. Each site's procedural guidelines specify the included services.

Surgery: Cardiovascular System— Codes 33010–37799

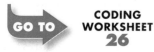

GO TO CODING WORKSHEET 26

The codes in this surgical subsection of CPT cover procedures performed on the cardiovascular system. Codes are grouped in two large sections, the heart and pericardium followed by the arteries and veins. Cardiac procedures include placement of pacemakers/pacing cardioverter defibrillators, surgery on the heart valves, and coronary artery bypass.

Many cardiac procedure codes include related procedures. For example, coronary artery bypasses include taking arteries or the saphenous vein graft from other body sites. Arterial and venous procedures, such as aneurysm repair, angioplasty, and catheter placement, include establishing blood inflow and outflow as well as arteriograms that the surgeon performs.

Internet Tip

The American College of Cardiology (ACC) is the association for physicians in the specialty of cardiology. As a service to its members, the ACC reports the addenda items that apply to their specialty each year. For example, access http://www.acc.org and explore the procedure coding updates related to cardiology. Report on how many new cardiology codes have been added for this year.

Surgery: Hemic and Lymphatic Systems; Mediastinum and Diaphragm— Codes 38100–39599

Codes in these two surgical subsections of CPT cover procedures involving the spleen, bone marrow or stem cell transplantation, lymph nodes and lymphatic channels, the mediastinum, and the diaphragm.

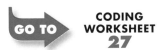

Coding Point

Surgical Procedures Include Diagnostic Procedures

As a general guideline, surgical procedures include diagnostic procedures. When a diagnostic procedure is the only service, it is reported. When the diagnostic procedure is followed by a surgical procedure, the diagnostic service is not reported. For example, a procedure such as a peritoneoscopy (laparoscopy examination of the peritoneum) to view and diagnose a condition is reported. However, if the diagnostic examination is followed by surgical laparoscopy (through the same scope and during the same surgical session), the diagnostic procedure cannot be separately reported. Note that a diagnostic laparoscopy as a separate procedure is located in the Digestive System subsection, code 49320.

GO TO **CODING WORKSHEET 27**

Surgery: Digestive System— Codes 40490–49999

The codes in the Digestive System surgical subsection of CPT cover procedures performed on the digestive system. Codes are grouped by body site: lips, mouth, pharynx, esophagus, stomach, intestines, rectum, anus, liver, biliary tract, pancreas, and abdomen. Each body site is organized by the type of procedure, such as excision and repair.

Endoscopic procedures are listed under the esophagus, intestines, rectum, anus, and biliary tract. In keeping with coding principles, the surgical endoscopic procedure includes the diagnostic endoscopic procedure.

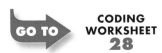

GO TO **CODING WORKSHEET 28**

Surgery: Urinary System— Codes 50010–53899

The codes in this surgical subsection of CPT cover procedures performed on the urinary system. Codes for the kidneys, ureters, bladder, and urethra are listed by the type of procedure. Different codes for males and females are indicated in some bladder and urethra procedures.

Many procedures involving the urinary system involve the use of a laparoscope or an endoscope. They include renal and ureteral laparoscopy and endoscopic procedures, cystoscopy (to view or treat the bladder), urethroscopy (to view or treat the urethra), and cystourethroscopy (using both the cystoscope and the urethroscope to view or treat the urinary collecting system). Therapeutic (surgical) procedures include diagnostic procedures as well as other listed procedures.

GO TO **CODING WORKSHEET 29A**

Surgery: Male Genital System; Intersex Surgery— Codes 54000–55980

The codes in the male genital system surgical subsection of CPT cover procedures performed on the male genital system. Codes for the penis, testis, epididymis, tunica vaginalis, scrotum, vas deferens, spermatic cord, seminal vesicles, and prostate are listed by type of procedure. Intersex codes cover male-to-female and female-to-male operative procedures.

GO TO **CODING WORKSHEET 29B**

Surgery: Female Genital System and Maternity Care/Delivery— Codes 56405–59899

The codes in these surgical subsections of CPT cover procedures performed on the female genital system and for maternity care and delivery. In the female genital system, codes for the vulva, perineum and introitus; vagina; cervix uteri; corpus uteri; oviduct/ovary; ovary; and for in vitro fertilization are listed by the type of procedure.

The maternity care and delivery codes have a unique organization. They are grouped as follows: antepartum (before birth) services; excision; introduction; repair; vaginal delivery, antepartum and postpartum (after birth) care; cesarean delivery; delivery after previous cesarean delivery; abortion; and other procedures.

The guidelines for maternity care/delivery describe the obstetric package of services normally provided for uncomplicated maternity cases. The package consists of antepartum care, delivery, and postpartum care, as described. Before coding obstetrical services, study these notes carefully to avoid unbundling—improperly reporting work that is part of the package. Understanding the obstetric package also permits correct reporting of those services that are not part of the package and that can be coded separately.

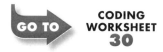

GO TO CODING WORKSHEET 30

Surgery: Endocrine System and Nervous System— Codes 60001–64999

The brief endocrine system subsection of the CPT Surgery section contains codes for procedure on the thyroid gland, parathyroid, thymus, adrenal glands, and carotid body.

The nervous system subsection has codes for nerves located in the skull, meninges, and brain; spine and spinal cord; extracranial nerves, peripheral nerves, and autonomic nervous system. Like the cardiovascular system section, the nervous system codes are complex, based on the particular anatomy and procedures required. Advances in techniques such as deep brain stimulation and pain management often lead to new and revised procedural codes in this section.

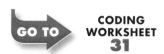

GO TO CODING WORKSHEET 31

Procedures Exempt from the -51 Modifier

In addition to add-on procedures or services, there are other procedures in CPT with which a -51 modifier for multiple surgical procedures cannot be used. The -51 modifier identifies additional surgical procedures that are done during the major, or primary, surgery. The primary procedure is paid in full, and the additional procedures automatically receive reduced payment (their Medicare RBRVS payment value has been reduced). Modifier -51 exempt codes are identified with the symbol ⊘.

Surgery: Eye and Ocular Adnexa; Auditory System; Operating Microscope— Codes 65091–69990

Codes in these subsections of CPT's Surgery section are used to report surgical procedures on the eye, its surrounding structures, and the ear. Ophthalmological diagnostic and treatment services are not coded from the Eye and Ocular Adnexa codes. Use the Ophthalmology codes in the Medicine section instead.

An operating microscope—code 69990— is used in the performance of delicate surgical procedures. In some cases, CPT permits reporting of the operating microscope; in other cases, its use is always part of the procedure, and it cannot be reported in addition to the operation. For example, a note at the beginning of the Eye and Ocular Adnexa Subsection states that the operating microscope should not be reported in addition to codes 65091 to 68850—that is, with all of the codes in this subsection. Be sure to review all notes when selecting codes.

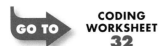

GO TO

CODING WORKSHEET 32

RADIOLOGY CODES

The codes in the Radiology section are used to report radiological services performed by or supervised by a physician. Radiology procedures have two parts:

1. *The technical component:* The technologist, the equipment, and processing, including preinjection and postinjection services such as local anesthesia, placement of needle or catheter, and injection of contrast material

2. *The professional component:* The reading of the radiological examination and the written report of interpretation by the physician

Radiology codes follow the same types of guidelines as noted in the Surgery section. For example, some radiology codes are identified as separate procedure codes. These codes are usually part of a larger, more complex procedure and should not be reported as separate codes unless the procedure was done independently. Also, some codes are add-on codes, such as those covering additional vessels that are studied after the basic examination. These codes are used with the primary codes, not alone.

Unlisted Procedures and Special Reports

New procedures are common in the area of radiology services. There are codes for nearly twenty unlisted code areas, such as:

78299   Unlisted gastrointestinal procedure, diagnostic nuclear medicine

When unlisted codes are reported, a special report must be attached that defines the nature, extent, and need for the procedure and describes the time, effort, and equipment necessary to provide it.

Contrast Material

For some radiological procedures, the physician decides whether it is best to perform the procedure with or without contrast material, a substance administered in the patient's blood vessels that helps highlight the area under study. For example, computerized tomography (CT) and magnetic resonance imaging (MRI) each provide different types of information about body parts and may be performed with or without contrast material. The term *with contrast* means only contrast materials given in the patient's veins or arteries. Contrast materials administered orally or rectally are coded as without contrast.

Structure and Modifiers

The diagnostic radiology, diagnostic ultrasound, and nuclear medicine subsections of the Radiology section are structured by type of procedure, followed by body sites and then specific procedures. For example:

Type: Diagnostic Ultrasound
Body site: Chest
Procedure: Echography, chest, B-scan and/or real time with image documentation

The radiation oncology subsection is organized somewhat differently. The first group of codes covers the planning services oncologists perform to set up a patient's radiation therapy treatment for cancer.

The following modifiers are commonly used in the Radiology section: -22, -26, -32, -51, -52, -53, -58, -59, -62, -66, -76, -77, -78, -79, -80, -90, and -99. Table 2.2 on pages 44–45 has a brief description of each modifier.

Assigning Radiology Codes

GO TO   CODING WORKSHEET 33

Most radiology services are performed and billed by radiologists working in hospital or clinic settings. Medical practices usually do not have radiology equipment and instead refer patients to these specialists. In many cases, the radiologist performs both the technical and the professional components.

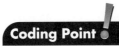

Coding Point

Modifier -26

If the physician does not own the equipment used for the radiology procedure, the modifier -26 is appended to the code, such as:

76511-26 Ophthalmic biometry by ultrasound echography, A-Scan

PATHOLOGY AND LABORATORY CODES

The codes in the Pathology and Laboratory section cover services provided by physicians or by technicians under the supervision of physicians. A complete procedure includes:

- Ordering the test
- Taking and handling the sample
- Performing the actual test
- Analyzing and reporting on the test results.

Panels

Certain tests are customarily ordered together to detect particular diseases or malfunctioning organs. These related tests are grouped under laboratory panels. When a panel code is reported, all the listed tests must have been performed. For example, the electrolyte panel requires these tests:

80051 Electrolyte panel
This panel must include the following:
Carbon dioxide (82374)
Chloride (82435)
Potassium (84132)
Sodium (84295)

Panels are considered bundled codes, so that if a panel code is reported, no individual test within it may be additionally reported. Other tests outside that panel may be reported if performed.

Structure and Modifiers

Procedures and services are listed in the Index under the following types of main terms:

- Name of the test, such as urinalysis, HIV, skin test
- Procedure, such as hormone assay
- Abbreviation, such as TLC screen
- Panel of tests, such as Complete Blood Count

The following modifiers are commonly used with pathology and laboratory codes: -22, -26, -32, -52, -53, -59, -90, and -91. Table 2.2 on pages 44–45 has a brief description of each modifier.

Assigning Pathology and Laboratory Codes

Some medical practices have laboratory equipment and perform their own testing. In-office labs are guided by federal safety regulations from OSHA (the Occupational Safety and Health Administration), and the tests that can be performed are regulated by CLIA (the Clinical Laboratory Improvement Amendment of 1988). The CLIA certification program awards one of three levels of certification. The lowest-level in-office certified lab can perform common tests, such as dipstick urinalysis and urine pregnancy.

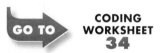
GO TO
CODING WORKSHEET 34

If the medical practice does not have an in-office lab, the physician may either take the specimen, reporting this service only (for example, using code 36415 for venipuncture to obtain a blood sample), and send it to an outside lab for processing or refer the patient to an outside lab for the complete procedure.

> ✓ **HIPAA Tip**
>
> **Laboratory Work**
>
> Medicare does not permit a physician who does not perform the lab work to bill for it. However, other payers permit this practice. When the physician orders the lab test and then pays the lab (called the reference lab) for the service, the physician may then report that test. The modifier -90 is attached to the code for the lab test.

MEDICINE CODES

The Medicine section contains the codes for the many types of evaluation, therapeutic, and diagnostic procedures that physicians perform. (Codes for the Evaluation and Management section described earlier, 99201 to 99499, fall numerically at the end of this section, but they appear first because they are the most frequently used codes.) Medicine codes may be used for procedures and services done or supervised by a physician of any specialty. They include many procedures and services provided by family practice physicians, such as immunizations and injections. The services of many specialists, such as allergists, cardiologists, and psychiatrists, are also covered in the Medicine section.

Codes from the Medicine section may be used with codes from any other section. Add-on codes and separate procedure codes are included in the Medicine section. Their use follows the guidelines described for previous sections. Unlisted procedure codes are provided for new procedures; a special report is required with unlisted codes.

Structure and Modifiers

The subsections are organized by type of service. Many subsections have notes containing usage guidelines and definitions. Some services, for example, have subcategories for new and established patients.

The following modifiers are commonly used with codes in the Medicine section: -22, -26, -32, -51, -52, -53, -55, -56, -57, -58, -59, -76, -77, -78, -79, -90, -91, and -99. Table 2.2 on pages 44–45 has a brief description of each modifier.

Assigning Medicine Codes

- Some of the services in the Medicine section are considered Evaluation and Management services, even though they are not listed in the E/M section. For these codes, the -51 modifier, Multiple Procedures, may not be used. For example, if a physician makes a second, brief visit to a patient in the hospital and also provides psychoanalysis, these services are reported separately:

  99231 Subsequent hospital care, problem focused/straightforward or low complexity decision making

  90845 Psychoanalysis

- Immunizations require two codes, one for administering the immunization and the other for the particular vaccine or toxoid that is given. For example, when a patient receives a MMRV vaccine, these two codes are used:

  90471 Immunization administration

  90710 Measles, mumps, rubella, and varicella vaccine (MMRV), live, for subcutaneous use

- The descriptors for injection codes also require two codes, one for the injection and one for the substance that is injected (the exception is allergy shots, which have their own codes in the Allergy and Clinical Immunology subsection). For example, to report the intravenous injection of erythromycin:

  90784 Therapeutic or diagnostic injection of erythromycin lactobionate; intravenous

  99070 Supplies and materials provided by the physician over and above those usually included in the office visit or other services rendered

For a Medicare patient, a HCPCS code is used for the material that is injected, instead of the general code 99070.

- Cardiac catheterizations are the most commonly performed surgical procedure; more than a million are performed each year. Complete coding of cardiac catheterization requires at least three codes: a code for the catheterization procedure itself, a code for the injection procedure, and a code for the imaging supervision and interpretation. Be aware that cardiac catheterizations—the catheter insertion and the imaging supervision and interpretation services, not the injection procedure—each have a professional and a technical component. Unless the physician owns the laboratory, those codes are billed with the -26 modifier.

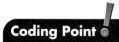

Coding Point

Immunizations and Office Visits

To report a patient's visit for just an immunization, some medical practices use E/M 99211 along with a code for the immunization. This is a misuse of the E/M code, which requires a significant, separate E/M service.

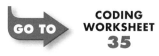

GO TO **CODING WORKSHEET 35**

CPT 2004 only © 2003 American Medical Association. All rights reserved.   Part 2: Coding Procedures   **73**

The Healthcare Common Procedure Coding System (HCPCS) is used to report procedures and services for Medicare patients and for most Medicaid claims. HCPCS has two code levels, referred to as Level I and Level II.

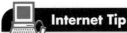
Internet Tip

Current HCPCS codes are available on the CMS Web site. Visit this location:
http://cms.hhs.gov/medicare/hcpcs/default.asp
and locate examples of temporary codes and effective dates for their use.

Level I Current Procedural Terminology

Level I repeats the CPT's five-number codes for physician procedures and services. Examples are:

99212   Office or other outpatient visit

00730   Anesthesia for procedures on upper posterior abdominal wall

24006   Arthrotomy of the elbow, with capsular excision for capsular release

70100   Radiologic examination of the mandible

80400   ACTH stimulation panel; for adrenal insufficiency

93000   Electrocardiogram, routine ECG with at least 12 leads; with interpretation and report

Level II National Codes

Level II is made up of more than 2,400 five-digit alphanumeric codes for items that are not listed in CPT. Most of these items are supplies, materials, or injections that are covered by Medicare. Some items are new services or procedures that are not covered in CPT.

Level II codes start with a letter followed by four digits, such as J7630. There are twenty-two sections, each covering a related group of items. For example, the E section covers the category of durable medical equipment (DME), reusable medical equipment ordered by the physician for use in the home, such as walkers and wheelchairs. The sections and code ranges are shown in Table 2.3. Examples are:

A0428   Ambulance service; basic life support, nonemergency

E0112   Crutches, underarm, wood, adjustable or fixed; pair, with pads, tips and handgrip

J0120   Injection, tetracycline, up to 250 mg

Table 2.3	HCPCS Level II Code Sections, Ranges, and Examples	
Section	**Code Range**	**Example**
Transportation services	A0000–A0999	A0300 Ambulance service; basic life support, nonemergency, all inclusive
Medical and surgical supplies	A4000–A7509	A4211 Supplies for self-administered injections
Miscellaneous and experimental	A9000–A9999	A9150 Nonprescription drugs
Enteral and parenteral therapy	B4000–B9999	B9000 Enteral nutrition infusion pump, without alarm
Temporary hospital Outpatient PPS	C0000 – C9999	C1170 Biopsy device, breast, abbi device
Dental procedures	D0000–D9999	D0150 Comprehensive oral exam
Durable medical equipment (DME)	E0000–E9999	E0250 Hospital bed with side rails and mattress
Procedures and services, temporary	G0000–G9999	G0001 Routine venipuncture for collection of specimen(s)
Rehabilitative services	H0000–H9999	H0006 Alcohol and/or drug services; case management
Drugs administered other than oral method	J0000–J8999	J0120 Injection, tetracycline, up to 250 mg
Chemotherapy drugs	J9000–J9999	J9212 Injection, interferon alfacon-1, recombinant, 1 mcg
Temporary codes for DMERCs*	K0000–K9999	K0001 Standard wheelchair
Orthotic procedures	L0000–L4999	L1800 Knee orthosis (KO); elastic with stays
Prosthetic procedures	L5000–L9999	L5050 Ankle, symes; molded socket, SACH foot
Medical services	M0000–M9999	M0064 Brief office visit for the sole purpose of monitoring or changing drug prescriptions used to treat mental psychoneurotic and personality disorders
Pathology and laboratory	P0000–P9999	P3000 Screening papanicolaou smear, cervical or vaginal, up to 3; by technician under physician supervision
Temporary codes	Q0000–Q0099	Q0034 Administration of influenza vaccine to Medicare beneficiaries by participating demonstration sites
Diagnostic radiology services	R0000–R5999	R0070 Transportation of portable X-ray equipment and personnel to home or nursing home, per trip to facility or location; one patient seen
Private payer codes	S0000–S9999	S0187 Tamoxifen citrate, oral, 10 mg
State Medicaid Agency Codes	T0000–T9999	T1001 Nursing assessment/evaluation
Vision services	V0000–V2999	V2020 Frames, purchases
Hearing services	V5000–V5999	V5364 Dysphagia screening

Source: HCPCS 2004

*DMERC=Durable Medical Equipment Regional Carriers

HCPCS Modifiers

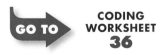

CODING WORKSHEET 36

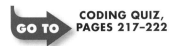

CODING QUIZ, PAGES 217–222

The two-letter modifiers that CMS developed for Medicare claims are useful indicators of other factors than those covered by CPT modifiers. For example, there are HCPCS modifiers for each finger and each toe. Because of their usefulness, many payers accept HCPCS modifiers in addition to CPT modifiers. The examples listed in Table 2.4 are the most commonly used.

CODING QUIZZES

The Coding Quizzes help you test your coding ability and practice your skills in working through certification examinations. You are ready to take the CPT Coding Quiz!

Table 2.4	Selected HCPCS Level II (National) Modifiers
Modifier	**Description**
-AA	Anesthesia services performed personally by anesthesiologist
-AB	Medical direction of own employee(s) by anesthesiologist (not more than four employees)
-AC	Medical direction of other than own employees by anesthesiologist (not more than four individuals)
-AG	Anesthesia for emergency surgery on a patient who is moribund or who has an incapacitating systemic disease that is a constant threat to life
-AH	Clinical psychologist
-AJ	Clinical social worker
-AM	Physician, team member service
-AS	Physician's assistant, nurse-practitioner, or clinical nurse specialist services for assistant at surgery
-BP	Beneficiary has been informed of the purchase/rental options; purchases the item
-BR	Beneficiary has been informed of the purchase/rental options; rents the item
-BU	Beneficiary has been informed of the purchase/rental options; has not informed supplier of decision after thirty days
-CC	Procedure change code (used to indicate a change in a submitted code)
-E1	Upper left, eyelid
-E2	Lower left, eyelid
-E3	Upper right, eyelid
-E4	Lower right, eyelid
-EJ	Subsequent claim for epoetin alfa-epo-injection claim
-FA	Left hand, thumb
-F1	Left hand, second digit
-F2	Left hand, third digit

Table 2.4	Selected HCPCS Level II (National) Modifiers, *continued*
Modifier	**Description**
-F3	Left hand, fourth digit
-F4	Left hand, fifth digit
-F5	Right hand, thumb
-F6	Right hand, second digit
-F7	Right hand, third digit
-F8	Right hand, fourth digit
-F9	Right hand, fifth digit
-GA	Waiver of liability statement on file
-GC	Service performed in part by resident under the direction of a teaching physician
-GX	Service not covered by Medicare
-LC	Left circumflex, coronary artery
-LD	Left anterior descending coronary artery
-RC	Right coronary artery
-LT	Left side (identifies procedures performed on the left side of the body)
-RT	Right side (identifies procedures performed on the right side of the body)
-QM	Ambulance service provided under arrangement by a provider of services
-QN	Ambulance service furnished directly by a provider of services
-QR	Repeat laboratory test performed on the same day
-TA	Left foot, great toe
-T1	Left foot, second digit
-T2	Left foot, third digit
-T3	Left foot, fourth digit
-T4	Left foot, fifth digit
-T5	Right foot, great toe
-T6	Right foot, second digit
-T7	Right foot, third digit
-T8	Right foot, fourth digit
-T9	Right foot, fifth digit
-TC	Technical component

Source: HCPCS 2004

● SUMMARY

1. CPT, a publication of the American Medical Association, contains the most widely used system of codes for physicians' medical, diagnostic, and procedural services. CPT codes are required for reporting physician practice services on insurance claims and encounter forms. The codes have five digits and a description. Updated versions are released annually. Medical practices must use the current codes because they can affect billing and reimbursement.

2. CPT contains six sections of codes, Evaluation and Management, Anesthesia, Surgery, Radiology, Pathology and Laboratory, and Medicine, followed by Category II and III codes, five appendixes, and an index. The index is used first in the process of selecting a code; it contains alphabetic descriptive main terms and subterms for the procedures and services contained in the main text. The codes themselves are listed in the main text and are generally grouped by body system or site or by type of procedure.

3. Each coding section begins with section guidelines, which discuss definitions and rules for the use of codes, such as for unlisted codes, special reports, and notes for specific subsections. When a main entry has more than one code, a semicolon follows the common part of a descriptor in the main entry, and the unique descriptors that are related to the common description are indented below it. Five symbols are used in the main text: (a) ● (a bullet or black circle) indicates a new procedure code; (b) ▲ (a triangle) indicates that the code's descriptor has changed; (c)► ◄ (facing triangles) enclose new or revised text other than the code's descriptor; (d) + (a plus sign) before a code indicates an add-on code that is used only along with other codes for primary procedures; and (e) a Ⓞ indicates that the code cannot be modified with a -51 modifier.

4. A CPT modifier is a two-digit number that may be attached to most five-digit procedure codes to indicate that the procedure is different from the listed descriptor, but not in a way that changes the definition or requires a different code. Two or more modifiers may be used with one code to give the most accurate description possible.

5. The first step in selecting a procedure code is to analyze the procedures and services to report by reviewing the documentation of the patient's visit. Next, after checking the coding system to use, CPT codes are located by finding the procedure in the index and verifying the code in the main text. The reporting order for the procedure codes places the code with the highest rate of reimbursement first. The final step is to determine whether modifiers are needed.

6. A summary of the six sections of codes follows:

SECTION	DEFINITION OF CODES	STRUCTURE	KEY GUIDELINES
Evaluation and Management	Physicians' services that are performed to determine the best course for patient care	Organized by place and/or type of service	New/established patients; other definitions Unlisted services/special reports Selecting an E/M service level
Anesthesia	Anesthesia services done by or supervised by a physician; includes general, regional, and local anesthesia	Organized by body site	Time-based Services covered (bundled) in codes Unlisted services/special reports Qualifying circumstances codes

SECTION	DEFINITION OF CODES	STRUCTURE	KEY GUIDELINES
Surgery	Surgical procedures performed by physicians	Organized by body system and then body site, followed by procedural groups	Surgical package definition Follow-up care definition Add-on codes Separate procedures Subsection notes Unlisted services/special reports Starred procedures
Radiology	Radiology services done by or supervised by a physician	Organized by type of procedure followed by body site	Unlisted services/special reports Supervision and interpretation (professional and technical components)
Pathology and Laboratory	Pathology and laboratory services done by physicians or by physician-supervised technicians	Organized by type of procedure	Complete procedure Panels Unlisted services/special reports
Medicine	Evaluation, therapeutic, and diagnostic procedures done or supervised by a physician	Organized by type of service or procedure	Subsection notes Multiple procedures reported separately Add-on codes Separate procedures Unlisted services/special reports

7. The key components for selecting Evaluation and Management codes are the extent of the history documented, the extent of the examination documented, and the complexity of the medical decision making. The steps for selecting correct E/M codes are to (a) determine the category and subcategory of service, (b) determine the extent of the history, (c) determine the extent of the examination, (d) determine the complexity of medical decision making, (e) analyze the requirements to report the service level, (f) verify the service level based on the nature of the presenting problem, time, counseling, and care coordination, (g) verify that the documentation is complete, and (h) assign the code.

8. HCPCS codes and modifiers are used primarily in the Medicare and Medicaid programs. There are two levels of codes. Level I repeats the codes in CPT. Level II, national codes, cover transportation, supplies, equipment, injections, and procedures not listed in CPT.

Coding Linkage and Compliance

Objectives

After studying this part, you will be able to:

1. Explain the importance of properly linking diagnoses and procedures when reporting services for reimbursement.
2. Discuss the major laws and guidelines that regulate coding compliance.
3. Describe actions that are considered fraudulent, and discuss the major types of errors medical practices make in reporting codes.
4. Explain the role of physician practice compliance plans and audits in avoiding fraud.
5. Apply key guidelines for coding compliance.

Key Terms

abuse	fraud	NCCI edits
assumption coding	Health Care Fraud and	Office of the Inspector
audit	Abuse Control Program	General (OIG)
code linkage	incident-to	OIG Work Plan
compliance plan	internal audit	*respondeat superior*
downcode	job reference aid	truncated coding
excluded parties	National Correct Coding	upcode
external audit	Initiative (NCCI)	

Why This Part Is Important to You

Physicians have the ultimate responsibility for proper documentation and correct coding, as well as for compliance with billing regulations. Health care claims, as well as the process used to create them, must comply with the rules imposed by federal and state law and with payer requirements. Correct coding helps reduce the chance of an investigation of the practice for improper billing, and the risk of liability if an investigation does occur.

The possible consequences of inaccurate coding and incorrect billing include

- Denied claims and reduced payments
- Delays in processing claims and receiving payments
- Fines and other sanctions; prison sentences
- Loss of hospital privileges
- Exclusion from payers' programs
- Loss of the physician's license to practice medicine

On correct claims, each reported service is connected to a diagnosis that supports the procedure as necessary to investigate or treat the patient's condition. Payers analyze this connection between the diagnostic and the procedural information, called **code linkage**, to evaluate the medical necessity of the reported charges. Correct claims also comply with other requirements, such as those dealing with the place or frequency of services.

This part of *Basic Medical Coding* gives you an understanding of correct, compliant coding practices. You will study key coding guidelines for avoiding fraud, and practice coding skills as you complete the Coding Worksheets and take the Coding Compliance Quiz.

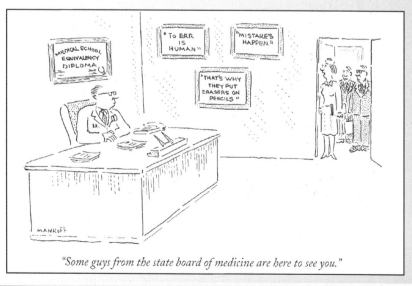

"Some guys from the state board of medicine are here to see you."

COMPLIANCE: AVOIDING FRAUD AND ABUSE

All medical staff must avoid any suggestion of fraudulent behavior in their work in physician practices. Almost everyone involved in the delivery of health care is a trustworthy person devoted to patients' welfare. However, some people are not. For example, according to the Department of Health and Human Services (HHS), in 2002 the federal government recovered more than $1.8 billion in judgments, settlements, and other fees in health care fraud cases.

Definitions of Fraud and Abuse

Fraud is an act of deception used to take advantage of another person or entity. For example, it is fraudulent for people to misrepresent their credentials or to forge another person's signature on a check. If a person pretends to be a physician and treats patients without a valid medical license, this is fraudulent. Fraudulent acts are intentional; they are made because the individual knows that some illegal or unauthorized benefit will probably result.

Claims fraud occurs when health care providers or others falsely represent their services or charges to payers. For example, a provider may bill for services that were not performed, code services at a higher level to increase payments, or fail to provide complete services under a contract. A patient may exaggerate an injury to get a settlement from an insurance company or ask medical office staff to change a date on a chart so that a service is covered by a health plan.

In federal law, **abuse** means an action that misuses the money that the government has allocated, such as Medicare funds. Abuse is illegal because taxpayers' dollars are misspent. An example of abuse is an ambulance service that billed Medicare for transporting a patient to the hospital when the patient did not need ambulance service. This abusive action resulted in improper payment for the ambulance company. In this example, the key difference between fraud and abuse is: to bill when the task was not done is fraud; to bill when it was not necessary is abuse.

Example

A billing manager for a plastic surgeons' group pleaded guilty to falsifying medical records to obtain insurance coverage for patients. She admitted that she falsified CT scan reports used to precertify insurance coverage for certain sinus-related surgeries. In some cases, when patients did not have serious enough underlying conditions to justify payment for surgery by insurance carriers, she falsified the report forms by cutting and pasting from her own personal CT scan report, which reflected a more serious underlying sinus condition. The billing manager faced a maximum sentence of eighteen months in prison and a criminal fine of up to $10,000, and had already agreed to pay $2,500 in civil insurance fraud fines as a condition of her plea.

Fraud and abuse charges are one of two types, according to the laws that apply. Most medical cases involve civil law, which regulates crimes against individuals' rights and the remedies for them. Examples of civil law cases are trespassing, divorce proceedings, and breach of contract. The punishment for those found guilty in a civil suit is typically a monetary fine. However, some cases of medical fraud and abuse involve criminal law. Criminal law typically regulates what are considered crimes against the state, such as kidnapping, robbery, and arson. The punishment for criminal acts is most often imprisonment as well as fines.

Example

Tenet Healthcare Corporation paid the federal government a record-setting $54 million as part of an ongoing criminal and civil investigation of alleged unnecessary cardiac procedures and surgeries at Redding Medical Center in California. The case involved allegations of unnecessary procedures, tests, lab studies, and surgeries. Tenet also agreed to random audits of cardiology procedures to be held twice yearly and other measures to ensure compliance.

Examples of Fraudulent or Abusive Acts

A number of actions are fraudulent or abusive. Investigators reviewing physicians' coding and billing work look for patterns like these:

- Reporting services that were not performed

    Example: A lab bills Medicare for a general health panel (CPT 80050), but the thyroid stimulating hormone (TSH) test was not done.

- Reporting services at a higher level than was carried out

    Example: After a visit for a flu shot, the provider bills the encounter as an Evaluation and Management service (CPT 99213) plus a vaccination (90471/90657).

- Performing and billing for procedures that are not related to the patient's condition and therefore not medically necessary

    Example: After reading an article about Lyme disease, a patient is worried about having worked in her garden over the summer, and she requests a Lyme disease diagnostic test. Although no symptoms or signs have been reported, the physician orders and bills for the Borrelia burgdorferi (Lyme disease) confirmatory immunoblot test (CPT 86617).

- Unbundling

    Example: When a primary care physician (PCP) orders a comprehensive metabolic panel (CPT 80053), the pathologist bills for the panel as well as for a quantitative glucose test (CPT 82947).

- Reporting the same service twice

    Example: On claims for a new patient who has been hospitalized for cardiac infarction, the cardiologist's office billed for initial observation care (CPT 99220) twice on the same date of service.

Coding compliance is a part of the overall effort of medical practices to comply with regulations in many areas. Medical practice staff as well as physicians must be aware of, understand, and comply with applicable regulations and laws.

Federal Law

A number of federal laws have made compliance with government regulations vital for medical practices. The two major laws are discussed below.

HIPAA Health Care Fraud and Abuse Control Program

HIPAA created the **Health Care Fraud and Abuse Control Program** to uncover fraud and abuse in the Medicare and Medicaid programs, as well as among private payers. Under this law, the **Office of the Inspector General (OIG)** has the task of detecting health care fraud and abuse and enforcing all laws relating to them.

OIG investigates suspected fraud cases and **audits** the records of physicians and third-party payers. In an audit, investigators review selected records for compliance with accepted documentation standards, such as the signing and dating of entries by the responsible health care professional and the linkage between the diagnosis and the procedures. The accounting records are often reviewed as well. When problems are found, the investigation proceeds and may result in charges of fraud or abuse against the practice.

Each year, as part of a Medicare Fraud and Abuse Initiative, the OIG announces the **OIG Work Plan**. The Work Plan lists the year's planned projects. To give you an idea of how the Work Plan relates to correct coding, read these points targeted in the 2004 Work Plan:

- *Consultations:* Determine the appropriateness of billings for physician consultation services and the financial impact of inaccurate billings on the Medicare program.

- *Coding of Evaluation and Management Services:* Examine whether physicians accurately coded Evaluation and Management services, for which Medicare paid over $23 billion in 2001.

- *Use of Modifier -25:* Determine whether providers used modifier -25 appropriately. In general, a provider should not bill evaluation and management codes on the same day as a procedure or other service unless the evaluation and management service is unrelated to such procedure or service. A provider reports such a circumstance by using modifier -25.

- *Services and supplies incident to physicians' services:* Evaluate the conditions under which physicians bill **incident-to** services and supplies. Physicians may bill for the services provided by allied health professionals, such as nurses, technicians, and therapists, as incident to their professional services. Incident-to services, which are paid at 100 percent of the Medicare physician fee schedule, must be provided by an employee of the physician under the physician's direct supervision.

If employees, physicians, and contractors such as coding/billing services have been found guilty of fraud, they may be excluded from work for government programs. An OIG exclusion has national scope and is important because Congress established a Civil Monetary Penalty for institutions that knowingly hire **excluded parties**. The OIG maintains the List of Excluded Individuals/Entities (LEIE), a database that provides the public, health care providers, patients, and others with information abut parties excluded from participation in Medicare, Medicaid, and federal health care programs.

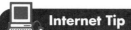

Internet Tip

Visit the OIG's Web site at

http://oig.hhs.gov/

to review the OIG Work Plan for either the current or the coming year.

Federal False Claims Act (31 USC § 3729)

The federal False Claims Act (FCA) prohibits submitting a fraudulent claim or making a false statement or representation in connection with a claim. It also encourages reporting of suspected fraud and abuse against the government by protecting and rewarding people involved in these cases.

Medicare Regulations

Medicare's national policy on correct coding is called the Medicare **National Correct Coding Initiative (NCCI)**. The NCCI is an ongoing process to standardize bundled codes and control improper coding that would lead to inappropriate payment for Medicare claims for physician services. The NCCI list contains more than two hundred thousand CPT code combinations. These code combinations, called **NCCI edits**, make up the computerized screening process used by Medicare to examine claims.

The NCCI edits determine what procedures and services cannot be billed together for the same patient on the same day of service. In the Medicare environment, these are billing errors—although they may be correctly coded.

There are three types of edits for NCCI errors:

- *Comprehensive versus component edits:* In this group, the first column of codes contains the comprehensive code, and the second column shows the component code. According to the NCCI, the comprehensive code includes all the services that are described by the component code, so the component code cannot be billed together with the comprehensive code for the same patient on the same day of service.

Example

Comprehensive   *Component*

27370   20610, 76000, 76003

- *Mutually exclusive edits:* This group also lists codes in two columns. According to CMS regulations, the services represented by these codes could not have both reasonably been done during a single patient encounter, so they cannot be billed together. If the provider reports both codes from both Column 1 and Column 2 for a patient on the same day, Medicare pays only the lower-paid code.

Example

Column 1   *Column 2*

50021   49061, 50020

- *Modifier indicators:* This type of NCCI modifier is a number appearing alongside the comprehensive and component code list and the mutually exclusive code list. A provider may include a NCCI modifier to allow payment for both services within the code pair under certain circumstances.

Internet Tip

Medicare NCCI Web Site

Visit the Web site that offers information and training on the National Correct Coding Initiative:

   http://cms.hhs.gov/medlearn/ncci.asp

Research the frequently asked questions about Correct Coding Principles and Edits to discover how often the NCCI edits are updated. To view the format of the NCCI edits as listed on the CMS Web site, visit

   http://cms.hhs.gov/physicians/cciedits/default.asp

Private Payer Regulations

Private payers develop code edits similar to the NCCI. Although private payers give medical practices information about their payment policies in their policy handbooks and bulletins, the exact code edits may not be shared with physicians. At times, their claims-editing software does not follow CPT guidelines and bundles distinct procedures or does not accept properly used modifiers. In these cases, medical office staff must follow up with the payer for clarification.

Policy handbooks usually contain additional regulations, such as the documentation required for certain procedures. Generally, the use of unlisted procedure codes requires a description of the services. Other services may also have special requirements. For example, a state Blue Cross and Blue Shield manual contains the requirement that the reporting of CPT code 90730, hepatitis A immunization, must be documented with the name of the serum, the dosage, and the route of administration.

GO TO   **CODING WORKSHEET 37**

Health care payers often base their decisions to pay or deny claims only on the diagnosis and procedure codes. The integrity of the request for payment rests on the accuracy and honesty of the coding. Incorrect coding may simply be an error, or it may represent deliberate efforts to obtain fraudulent payment. Some compliance errors are related to medical necessity; others are a result of incorrect code selection or billing practices.

Errors Relating to Code Linkage and Medical Necessity

To establish medical necessity, the payer must understand the severity of the patient's condition and the signs, symptoms, or history that relate to the reason for care. To be appropriately linked diagnosis and procedure codes must pass the test of clinical consistency. For example, if a condition has been diagnosed, other reported symptoms must be related to it—shortness of breath should have a logical primary diagnosis, such as lung disease, heart failure, or anxiety. Treatments should be related to functional impairments and disabilities. And clinically, the overall coding of the case should be reasonable. These facts must be documented in the patient's medical record as well as in the codes.

Claims are denied due to lack of medical necessity when the reported services are not consistent with the symptoms/diagnosis or not in keeping with generally accepted professional medical standards. Correctly linked codes that support medical necessity meet these conditions:

- The CPT procedure codes match the ICD-9-CM diagnosis codes.

Example: A procedure to drain an abscess of the external ear or auditory canal should be supported by a diagnosis of disorders of the external ear or an ear carbuncle or cyst.

- The procedures are not elective, experimental, or nonessential.

Example: Cosmetic nasal surgery performed to improve a patient's appearance is typically excluded. However, a cosmetic procedure may be considered medically necessary when it is performed to repair an accidental injury or to improve the functioning of a malformed body member. A diagnosis of deviated septum, nasal obstruction, acquired facial deformity, or the late effects of facial bone fracture supports the medical necessity for cosmetic nasal surgery.

- The procedures are furnished at an appropriate level.

Example: A high-level Evaluation and Management code for an office visit (such as 99204/99205 and 99214/99215) must be matched by a serious, complex condition such as a sudden, unexplained large loss of weight.

Errors Relating to the Coding Process

To avoid coding errors, it is essential that all codes are currently correct and complete. **Truncated coding**, in which diagnosis codes are not reported at the highest level of specificity available, causes rejected claims, as does using codes that are out of date. The gender or age of the patient must match the selected code when the code involves selection for either criterion. Documentation must clearly support the codes. Following are other incorrect practices:

- **Assumption coding**—reporting items or services that are not actually documented, but that the coder assumes were performed
- Altering documentation after services are reported
- Coding without proper documentation
- Reporting services provided by unlicensed or unqualified clinical personnel
- Not having all necessary documentation available at the time of coding
- Not satisfying the conditions of coverage for a particular service, such as the physician's direct supervision of a radiologist's work
- Not complying with the billing requirements for a service, such as the rules for global surgical period coverage.

Errors Relating to the Billing Process

A number of errors are related to the billing process. These errors include reporting services that are not covered or have limited coverage, and using modifiers incorrectly. Another error involvces **upcoding**—using a procedure code that provides a higher reimbursement rate than the code that actually reflects the service provided. When upcoding is found by the payer, the code is changed to a lower-value code that the payer thinks is correct. This action is called **downcoding**.

Unbundling—billing the parts of a bundled procedure as separate procedures—must also be avoided. For clarity on the procedures that bundled surgical codes contain, medical practices should be specific about their descriptions of these codes. Many practices adopt Medicare's NCCI list of bundling rules for such codes, and others adopt the slightly different list from the American Medical Association. Practices communicate their standard to the private payers with whom they work.

THE COMPLIANCE PLAN

For medical coders, strategies for avoiding fraud and abuse are especially important. This can be a difficult and complex assignment. Coding claims in order to generate payment at the highest appropriate level is a critical goal of the coding and billing staff's responsibilities. Sometimes, however, regulations can be unclear or even disagree with each other. There are two types of strategies. The first, the compliance plan, is at the practice level. The second involves measures coders take in their day-to-day work to prevent problems.

Because of the risk of fraud and abuse liability, medical practices must be sure that regulations are followed by all staff members. In addition to responsibility for their own actions, physicians are liable for the professional actions of employees they supervise. This responsibility is a result of the law of *respondeat superior*, which states that an employer is responsible for an employee's actions. Physicians are held to this doctrine, so they can be charged for the fraudulent behavior of any staff member.

A wise slogan is, "the best defense is a good offense." For this reason, a medical practice creates and implements a **compliance plan** to find compliance problems and correct them to avoid risking liability. A compliance plan is a written plan describing how the practice will (1) audit and monitor compliance with government regulations, especially in the area of coding and billing, (2) develop written policies and procedures that are consistent, (3) provide for ongoing staff training and communication, and (4) respond to and correct errors.

Compliance Guideline

Medical Liability Insurance

Medical liability cases for fraud often result in lawsuits. Professional liability insurance is purchased by physicians to cover such legal expenses. Although covered under the physician's policy, other medical professionals often purchase their own liability insurance. Medical coders are also advised to have professional liability insurance called error and omission (E&O) insurance, which protects against financial loss due to intentional or unintentional failure to perform work correctly.

Auditing

Compliance audits judge whether the practice's physicians and coding and billing staff comply with regulations for correct coding and billing. An audit does not involve reviewing every claim and document. Instead, a representative sample is studied to reveal whether erroneous or fraudulent behavior exists. If the auditor finds indications of a problem on the sample, more documents and more detail are usually reviewed.

For example, a practice that reported only the top two of a five-level E/M code range for new or established patient office visits would not fit a normal pattern of office visit codes. The normal pattern has codes at all levels, with more codes in the middle and fewer at the first and the fifth levels. While reporting outside of the normal range is sometimes justified by a practice's circumstances, most often it is evidence of a compliance problem.

In an **external audit**, private payers' or government investigators review selected records of a practice for compliance. Coding linkage, completeness of documentation, and adherence to documentation standards, such as the signing and dating of entries by the responsible health care professional, may all be studied. The accounting records are often reviewed as well.

To reduce the chance of an investigation or external audit and to reduce potential liability when one occurs, most practices' compliance plans require **internal audits** to be conducted regularly, either by the medical practice staff or by a hired consultant. These audits are routine and are performed periodically without a reason to think that a compliance problem exists. They help the practice determine whether coding is being done appropriately and whether all performed services are being reported for maximum revenue and documented.

Ongoing Training

Part of the compliance plan is a commitment to keep physicians trained in pertinent coding and regulatory matters. Medical office staff—often a coder—train physicians on changed codes or medical necessity regulations. The following guidelines are helpful in conducting physician training classes:

- Keep the presentation as brief and straightforward as possible.
- In a multispecialty practice, issues should be discussed by specialty; all physicians do not need to know changed rules on dermatology, for example.
- Use actual examples, and stick to the facts when presenting material.
- Explain the benefits of coding compliance to the physicians, and listen to their feedback to improve job performance.
- Set up a way to address additional changes during the year, such as an office newsletter or compliance meetings.

Ongoing training also requires having the current annual updates, reading health plans' bulletins and periodicals, and researching changed regulations.

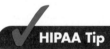

HIPAA Tip

Keeping Previous Code Books

When new updates for the ICD-9-CM and CPT codes are received, the previous year's code books should be retained in the event of a question or investigation of claims from prior years.

Correct Preparation of Job Reference Aids

Many medical practices develop **job reference aids**, also known as cheat sheets, to help the coding process. These aids usually list the procedures and CPT codes that are most frequently reported by the practice. Some also list frequently used diagnoses with ICD codes. Although job reference aids can be helpful during the coding process, they may also lead to questions about compliance. Are codes assigned by selecting one that is close to the patient's condition on the aid, rather than by researching the precise code based on the documentation?

If job reference aids are used in a practice, these guidelines should be followed:

- Job reference aids should be dated, to be sure that current codes are in use, and reissued every year with updated codes.

- The job reference aid for CPT codes must contain all the codes in a range that the practice may assign. For example, if the medical practice includes office visit codes on a CPT aid, all ten codes should be listed (five levels for both new and established patients).

- An aid for ICD-9-CM codes should be presented in one of two ways. (1) The aid should have only the ICD categories (three-digit numbers) to speed the code selection process; and the manual should be reviewed for the proper usage and highest degree of specificity. (2) If three-, four-, and five-digit codes are listed, the complete range should be shown, not one or two codes from the group. For example, if heartburn is to be listed, the complete range of symptoms involving the digestive system (787.0–787.99) should be shown, with the correct level of specificity shown as well.

Many practices also list CPT and ICD-9-CM codes on the office's encounter form. In some cases, these are the only codes listed; in others, these standard codes are shown next to the accounting codes the practice uses. Encounter forms, like job reference aids, must not select from various codes in a range; all the possibilities should be listed, so that it is clear that all have been considered before the code is checked on the encounter form.

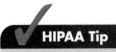

HIPAA Tip

Compliant Job Reference Aids

Job reference aids or encounter forms should never link diagnoses and procedures. This practice gives the appearance that coding is based on reimbursement rather than on the patient's condition.

GO TO

CODING WORKSHEET 38

Internet Tip

The American Compliance Institute provides a forum for compliance officers to exchange information on compliance-related issues. Visit

http://www.compliance.com

and research this site. What types of publications and newsletters are available?

For medical office staff, the best defense against fraud investigations is to prevent them from happening in the first place. These measures help prevent problems:

- Keep coding knowledge up to date through ongoing continuing education in changing codes
- Read payer bulletins and regulatory publications, and update the written policies and procedures
- Review coding accuracy by asking:

    Do the diagnosis codes relate correctly to the procedure codes?

    Are reported codes supported by documentation in the patient medical record?

    Are there any unusual coding patterns, such as using only the highest reimbursement level of codes rather than the expected range of levels?

    Has the proper code set, such as HCPCS codes as applicable for Medicare patients, been used?

- File all written correspondence with government-sponsored and other payers, and be sure that any recommendations from them on billing matters are in writing
- Clarify coding and billing questions with physicians, and be sure that the physician adds any needed clarification to the documentation
- Use the information from claims that are denied or paid at a lesser rate to modify procedures as needed

Following are specific tips to follow to code compliantly. After reading each tip, complete the Coding Worksheet to check your understanding.

Verifying Linkage

Appropriately linked diagnosis and procedure codes pass the test of clinical consistency. When a condition has been diagnosed, other reported conditions and/or symptoms must be related to it, and treatments should be related to functional impairments and disabilities. For CPT evaluation and management (E/M) codes, the diagnosis code should support the level of the E/M code. For example, a diagnosis of dermatitis due to sunburn does not support the medical necessity of a comprehensive examination, even if the physician performs and documents all required components. For procedures, the diagnosis code should relate clinically to the procedure. Clinically, then, the overall coding of the case should be reasonable.

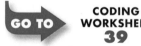

GO TO
**CODING
WORKSHEET
39**

Selecting the Primary Diagnosis

The primary diagnosis, or condition, is the most important reason for the care provided. It is reported first, if more than one condition is pertinent or treated. Additional codes are listed to describe all documented, current coexisting conditions that affect patient treatment or require treatment during the encounter. Coexisting conditions may be related to the primary diagnosis, or they may involve a separate illness that the physician diagnoses and treats during the encounter. Only the definitive condition or conditions that caused the encounter are coded. Symptoms that are integral to a diagnosis, such as stomach pain related to bowel obstruction, are not reported.

Some conditions require the assignment of two codes. A code may be needed for the disease's etiology and another for its manifestation, or typical signs or symptoms. Manifestation codes are shown in italics in the ICD-9-CM and are never primary, even when the diagnostic statement is written in that order. In some cases, a combination code may cover both etiology and manifestation.

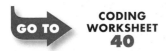
GO TO CODING WORKSHEET 40

Reporting Chronic or Undiagnosed Conditions

A chronic condition—one that continues over a long period of time or recurs frequently—is reported each time the patient receives care for that condition. However, conditions that are no longer being treated or no longer exist are not reported, unless the documentation shows that a previous history is pertinent to the current condition. Some encounters cover both an acute and a chronic condition. If both the acute and the chronic illnesses are treated and each has a code, list the acute code first.

Diagnoses are not always established at the first encounter. In this case, diagnosis codes that cover symptoms, signs, and ill-defined conditions are used. Inconclusive diagnoses, such as those preceded by "rule out," "suspected," or "probable," are not coded. Code only to the highest degree of certainty, listing the most definitive diagnosis first.

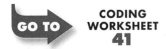
GO TO CODING WORKSHEET 41

Using V and E Codes for a Clear Picture of an Encounter

V codes, for factors influencing health status and contact with health services, and E codes, for external causes of injury and poisoning, are often required to provide a complete picture of the medical necessity for reported procedures. These codes may also help establish liability among payers, such as primary medical insurance and workers' compensation coverage.

Some V codes, such as those for general medical examinations and screening tests, are used as primary diagnoses. Others, such as V codes for a family or personal history of a disease, may not be used as primary; rather, they are listed as secondary codes. E codes are always secondary to the primary diagnosis, because their purpose is to describe a cause, not a condition or a reason for an encounter.

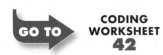
GO TO CODING WORKSHEET 42

Avoiding Unspecified Diagnosis Codes

Unspecified diagnosis codes—usually those that end in 0 or 9 within a category—indicate that a particular body site was not documented, although classifications are available, or other information is not present. The lack of information causes selection of an unspecified code that may not prove medical necessity, because it is considered too vague to support the requirement for the procedure. When documentation is insufficient, often coders request more specific information.

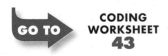
GO TO CODING WORKSHEET 43

Reporting Surgical Diagnoses and Complications

When surgery is performed and the preoperative diagnosis changes, the new postoperative diagnosis code is reported, rather than the preoperative code.

If complications arise during the procedure, the primary diagnosis is the first code reported. The complication is coded in addition, following the primary diagnosis. However, if the complications arise after the procedure is complete and require an additional procedure, the complication is the primary diagnosis for the later procedure. Many complications of surgical and medical care are contained in categories 996–999.

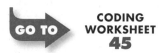

GO TO CODING WORKSHEET 44

Reporting Bundled (Global) Procedures and Laboratory Panels

Unbundling—reporting procedures that are covered under another code as additional work—of surgical codes and of laboratory panels is non-compliant. A careful reading of the section notes and procedural descriptors in CPT indicates which procedures are included in various codes.

General principles also apply. For example, surgical procedures always include the diagnostic procedures that precede them (on the same day of service). An application of this point is the fact that when a biopsy precedes the excision of a lesion, only the excision is reported.

It is also important to review the individual tests that comprise each laboratory panel. Multiple panels are often ordered. If the component tests overlap, only one panel is reported, along with the differing individual tests from the other panels.

GO TO CODING WORKSHEET 45

CODING QUIZZES

The Coding Quizzes help you test your coding ability and practice your skills in working through certification examinations. You are ready to take the Coding Linkage and Compliance Quiz!

GO TO CODING QUIZ, PAGES 223–225

SUMMARY

1. Diagnoses and procedures must be correctly linked when services are reported for reimbursement, because payers analyze this connection to determine the medical necessity of the charges. Correct claims also comply with all applicable regulations and requirements. Codes should be appropriate and documented as well as compliant with each payer's rules.

2. The major laws and guidelines that regulate coding compliance include (a) federal laws, such as the Health Care Fraud and Abuse Control Program and the False Claims Act (FCA); (b) the annual OIG Work Plan that pursues the goals of the Medicare Fraud and Abuse Initiative; (c) national Medicare regulations and code edits contained in the NCCI and local carriers' rules; and (d) private payers' code edits and regulations.

3. A number of actions are considered fraudulent when they are part of a repeated pattern, such as reporting services that were not performed, reporting at a higher level than performed, billing for procedures that were not medically necessary to treat the patient's condition, unbundling services, and repeat billing for the same service. Claims are rejected or downcoded because of (a) medical necessity errors, including poor linkage between procedures and conditions, services at an inappropriate level, and billing for experimental procedures; (b) coding errors, such as truncated diagnosis codes and codes that lack proper documentation; and (c) errors related to billing, such as reporting uncovered services, using incorrect modifiers, and upcoding.

4. A physician practice compliance plan describes how the practice will (1) audit and monitor compliance with government regulations, especially in the area of coding and billing, (2) develop written policies and procedures that are consistent, (3) provide for ongoing staff training and communication, and (4) respond to and correct errors. External audits are conducted by private or government payers to ensure practice compliance with coding and billing regulations. Internal audits help the practice reduce the possibility that claims will be rejected or downcoded due to coding compliance errors.

5. Key guidelines for coding compliance include using correct job reference aids, verifying code linkage, selecting the primary diagnoses, correctly coding chronic/undiagnosed conditions, using V and E codes to clearly describe encounters, avoiding the use of unspecified diagnosis codes, correctly coding surgical complications, and avoiding unbundling of global procedure codes and laboratory panels.

PART 4

Coding Worksheets

Alphabetic Index and Tabular List

Answer these questions about the ICD-9-CM Alphabetic Index:

1. The following entry appears in the Alphabetic Index of the ICD.

   Kimmelstiel(-Wilson) disease or syndrome
   (Intercapillary glomerulosclerosis) 250.4 *[581.81]*

   What type of term is *Kimmelstiel(-Wilson)?*

   _____

   What type of term is shown indented and in parentheses?

   _____

   Does this disease require one or two codes?

   _____

2. Locate the following main terms. List and interpret any cross-references you find next to the entries.

   La grippe _____

   Anginoid pain _____

   Branchial _____

3. Are *see* cross-references in the Alphabetic Index followed by codes? Why?

   _____

4. Locate the main term Choledocholithiasis, and explain the purpose of the note beneath it.

   _____

Provide the following information about codes found in the Tabular List.

5. What agent is excluded from subcategory 972.0, cardiac rhythm regulators?

   _____

6. A brace is located under 562.00. What does the brace mean?

   _____

7. What is the meaning of the symbol in front of category 017?

   _____

8. What types of gastric ulcers are included in category 531?

   _____

9. What is the meaning of the phrase that follows subclassification 466.19?

   _____

10. What is the meaning of the phrase that follows subcategory 730.7?

   _____

11. Place a double underline below the main terms and a single underline below any subterms in each of the following statements, and then determine the correct codes.

A. cerebral atherosclerosis _____

B. spasmodic asthma with status asthmaticus _____

C. congenital night blindness _____

D. recurrent inguinal hernia with obstruction _____

E. incomplete bundle branch heart block _____

F. acute bacterial food poisoning _____

G. malnutrition following gastrointestinal surgery _____

H. skin test for hypersensitivity _____

I. frequency of urination at night _____

V Codes and E Codes

Provide the V code for the following encounters.

1. routine medical examination _____

2. exposure to tuberculosis _____

3. glaucoma screening _____

4. supervision of high-risk first pregnancy in a 15-year-old female _____

5. measles vaccination _____

6. admission for prophylactic removal of ovary _____

7. attention to cleansing of ureterostomy _____

8. heart transplant (status post) _____

9. diaphragm fitting _____

10. exposure to lead _____

11. family history of polycystic kidney disease _____

12. inoculation against diphtheria _____

13. annual checkup of 8-year-old girl _____

14. screening of fetus by amniocentesis _____

15. delivery of live twin infants, mother's record _____

16. replacement with artificial knee _____

17. fitting of artificial eye _____

18. counseling a neglected child _____

19. encounter with kidney donor _____

20. patient seeking counseling for loss of spouse _____

21. follow-up encounter after chemotherapy _____

22. Papanicolaou smear and annual pelvic examination _____

23. adjustment of hearing aid _____

24. encounter for occupational therapy _____

25. status of tracheostomy _____

For the following encounters, provide the V code and indicate whether it is a primary or a supplemental code.

26. preoperative cardiovascular examination _____

27. encounter for hospice care _____

28. health examination of preschool children _____

29. counseling for marital problems _____

30. supervision of normal first pregnancy _____

31. patient's parents are both deaf _____

32. history of allergy to dust _____

33. patient suspected of carrying hepatitis C _____

34. infection with penicillin-resistant microorganism _____

35. encounter for suture removal _____

Identify the E codes for the following substances in the Table of Drugs and Chemicals.

1. accidental poisoning by barbiturates _____

2. accidental poisoning by malathion _____

3. injury from ingesting Oestriol _____

4. suicide attempt with aspirin _____

5. adverse effect from diphtheria vaccine _____

Provide the E codes for the following descriptions.

6. accidental drowning after fall from water skis _____

7. fall from a window _____

8. sunstroke _____

9. bee sting _____

10. injury to driver in motor vehicle collision with a stalled car _____

11. passenger in snowmobile injured in fall _____

12. injury to airplane pilot during a crash while landing _____

13. glue use in a suicide attempt _____

14. accidental poisoning with Mercurochrome _____

15. suffocation due to blockage of air passages by food _____

16. patient struck on the head by a falling tree _____

17. patient accidentally injured by unsterile procedure during kidney dialysis _____

18. fall on an escalator _____

19. cuts caused by broken glass _____

20. patient injured by a horse kick _____

21. wounds from a battle in a war _____

22. assault by nerve gas _____

23. adverse reaction to an aspirin taken for a headache _____

24. bicycle rider injured in accidental fall _____

25. headache resulting from combined estrogen and progestogen, daily dosage _____

26. exposure to radiation _____

27. burn caused by flames of gas grill in kitchen _____

28. railway passenger injured while boarding the train _____

29. adverse reaction to anti-parkinsonism drug _____

30. injury during a hurricane _____

For the following descriptions, provide both the primary code for the patient's diagnosis and the supplemental E code in the correct order.

31. allergic reaction to synthetic penicillin *Hint:* First code the allergic reaction and then code the adverse reaction to the therapeutic use. _____

32. fractured thumb on right hand resulting from a fall from a ladder _____

33. dermatitis due to an adverse reaction to antihistamine _____

34. patient tackled and knocked down during football game, suffers concussion with brief loss of consciousness _____

35. coma caused by overdose of tranquilizers in suicide attempt _____

Working with the ICD-9-CM

Section A

Why is it important to use the Alphabetic Index and then the Tabular List to find the correct code? Work through this coding process, and then comment on your result.

> Double-underline the main term and underline the subterm.
>> patient complains of abdominal cramps

> Find the term in the Alphabetic Index, and list its code.

> _____

> Verify the code in the Tabular List, reading all instructions. List the code you have determined to be correct.

> _____

> Did the result of your research in the Tabular List match the main term's code in the Alphabetic Index? Why?

> _____

Section B

Match the key terms with the correct definitions.

   A. E code
   B. unspecified
   C. Tabular List
   D. category
   E. V code
   F. manifestation
   G. eponym
   H. convention
   I. main term
   J. supplementary term

_____ 1. Typographic technique or standard practice that provides visual guidelines for understanding printed material

_____ 2. The medical term in boldfaced type that identifies a disease or condition in the Alphabetic Index

_____ 3. An alphanumeric code used to identify the external cause of an injury or poisoning

_____ 4. A nonessential word or phrase that helps define a diagnosis code

_____ **5.** The part of the ICD-9-CM that contains chapters with code categories

_____ **6.** Refers to a code that should be used for an incompletely described condition

_____ **7.** An alphanumeric code used for an encounter that is not due to illness or injury

_____ **8.** A three-digit code that covers a single disease or related condition

_____ **9.** The characteristic signs or symptoms associated with a disease

_____ **10.** A condition or procedure that is named for the physician who discovered it

Section C

Decide whether each statement is true or false, and write T for true or F for false.

_____ **1.** In selecting correct diagnosis codes, the chapters of the Tabular List are first searched, and the code is then verified in the Alphabetic Index.

_____ **2.** Subcategories are four-digit diagnosis codes that define the etiology, site, or manifestation of a disease.

_____ **3.** In the Alphabetic Index, a _see_ cross-reference must be followed.

_____ **4.** The etiology of a disease refers to the reason that the patient presents for treatment.

_____ **5.** The fifth-digit requirement refers to the need to show a subclassification code for a particular diagnosis.

_____ **6.** A code that appears in italics is a secondary code and is not sequenced first.

_____ **7.** The coding instruction "use an additional code" means that supplying another code is optional.

_____ **8.** A patient has an appointment for a complaint of flulike symptoms. While the patient is in the office, the physician decides to conduct a complete physical examination. A V code is used as the primary diagnosis code for the encounter.

_____ **9.** When a diagnosis is being confirmed by tests or other procedures, only the patient's signs, symptoms, or vague condition are coded, not the possible or suspected disease.

_____ **10.** A patient's past, cured conditions have no applicability to the coding of current encounters except when late effects are noted.

Section D

Write the letter of the choice that best completes the statement or answers the question.

____ **1.** Outpatient coding is based on which volume or volumes of the ICD-9-CM?

    A. Volume 1
    B. Volumes 1 and 2
    C. Volumes 1, 2, and 3
    D. Volumes 2 and 3

____ **2.** The medical terms in the Alphabetical Index are arranged by

    A. the condition or problem
    B. the anatomical site
    C. the etiology and the manifestation
    D. the signs and symptoms

____ **3.** The unintentional, harmful reaction to a correct dosage of a drug is called

    A. a late effect
    B. a coexisting condition
    C. an adverse effect
    D. a manifestation

____ **4.** A condition that remains or recurs after an acute illness has finished is called

    A. a late effect
    B. a coexisting condition
    C. an adverse effect
    D. a manifestation

____ **5.** A colon after a term in an *excludes* or *includes* note indicates that

    A. the term is not complete without one or more of the additional terms listed
    B. the term requires a manifestation code
    C. the synonyms, alternative wordings, or explanations that follow may appear in the diagnostic statement
    D. the term requires a code for the underlying disease

____ **6.** To code an encounter for chemotherapy, list the codes in the following order:

    A. E code, condition code
    B. condition code, E code
    C. V code, condition code
    D. condition code, V code

_____ **7.** The diagnostic statement "patient presents for removal of a cast" requires the use of which of the following types of codes?

    A. E

    B. V

    C. R

    D. M

_____ **8.** If a patient is treated for both an acute and a chronic condition, each of which has a separate code, how should the codes be listed?

    A. V code, condition code

    B. chronic code, acute code

    C. acute code, V code

    D. acute code, chronic code

Practice ICD Coding

Section A

Supply the correct ICD-9-CM codes for the following diagnoses.

1. Brewer's infarct _____
2. conjunctivitis due to Reiter's disease _____
3. seasonal allergic rhinitis due to pollen _____
4. cardiac arrhythmia _____
5. backache _____
6. sebaceous cyst _____
7. breast disease, cystic _____
8. chronic cystitis _____
9. normal delivery _____
10. skin tags _____
11. acute myocarditis due to influenza _____
12. acute otitis media _____
13. endocarditis due to Q fever _____
14. influenza vaccination _____
15. vertigo _____
16. essential anemia _____
17. muscle spasms _____
18. influenza with acute respiratory infection _____
19. pneumonia due to Streptococcus, Group B _____
20. menorrhagia _____

Section B

Provide the diagnostic code(s) for the following cases, and explain the coding guideline that you applied to the case.

1. A thirty-six-year-old female patient presents to the physician's office for her yearly checkup. During the exam, the physician identifies a palpable, solitary lump in the left breast. The physician considers this significant and extends the exam to gather information for diagnosing this problem.

   _____

2. A forty-five-year-old male patient presents to the office complaining of headaches for the past twenty-four hours. Based on the examination, the physician orders an MRI to investigate a possible brain tumor.

   _____

3. An eighty-six-year-old female patient who has a chronic laryngeal ulcer presents for treatment of a painful episode.

_____

4. A fifty-eight-year-old female patient has muscle weakness due to poliomyelitis in childhood.

_____

5. A sixty-four-year-old male patient's diagnosis is degenerative osteoarthritis.

_____

Section C

Audit the following cases to determine if the correct codes have been reported in the correct order. If a coding mistake has been made, state the correct code and your reason for assigning it.

1. Chart note for Henry Blum, date of birth 11/4/53:
Examined patient on 12/6/2006. He was complaining of a facial rash. Examination revealed sebopsoriasis and extensive seborrheic dermatitis over his upper eyebrows, nasolabial fold, and extending to the subnasal region.

The following codes were reported: 696.1, 690.1.

_____

2. Physician's notes, 2/24/2005, patient George Kadar, DOB 10/11/1940:
Subjective: This sixty-four-year-old patient complains of voiding difficulties, primarily urinary incontinence. No complaints of urinary retention.
Objective: Rectal examination: enlarged prostate. Patient catheterized for residual urine of 200 cc. Urinalysis is essentially negative.
Assessment: Prostatic hypertrophy, benign.
Plan: Refer to urologist for cystoscopy.

The following code was reported: 600.0.

_____

3. An insulin-dependent diabetic patient is seen for a blood glucose screening.

The following codes were reported: 250.01, V77.1.

_____

4. Patient: Gloria S. Diaz
Subjective: This twenty-five-year-old female patient presents with pain in her left knee both when she moves it and when it is inactive. She denies previous trauma to this area but has had right-knee pain and arthritis in the past.
Objective: Examination revealed the left knee to be warm and slightly swollen compared to the right knee. Extension is 180 degrees; flexion is 90 degrees. Some tenderness in area.
Assessment: Left-knee pain probably due to chronic arthritis.
Plan: Daypro 600 mg 2-QD x 1 week; recheck in one week.

The following codes were reported: 719.48, 716.98.

_____

Infectious and Parasitic Diseases

Provide the codes for the following diagnoses.

1. trichinosis _____

2. trichuriasis _____

3. Lyme disease _____

4. tabes dorsalis _____

5. ECHO virus _____

6. ovale malaria _____

7. Behcet's syndrome _____

8. primary genital syphilis _____

9. viral hepatitis A without mention of hepatic coma _____

10. rabies _____

11. postmeasles pneumonia _____

12. AIDS _____

13. enteritis due to astrovirus _____

14. botulism _____

15. roundworm infection _____

16. candidal onychia _____

17. swimmer's itch _____

18. sand flea infestation _____

19. Rocky Mountain spotted fever _____

20. mumps with hepatitis _____

21. venereal verruca _____

22. Coxsackie pericarditis _____

23. ambulatory plague _____

24. Staphylococcus aureus septicemia _____

25. scarlatina anginosa _____

26. tuberculous laryngitis, bacteriological examination not done _____

For the following descriptions, check the "Include" note when assigning the code.

27. chronic hepatitis E without mention of hepatic coma _____

28. Malta fever _____

29. amebic skin ulceration due to Entamoeba histolytica _____

30. chronic gonococcal cystitis _____

31. recurrent tick-borne fever _____

32. pertussis due to Bordetella bronchiseptica _____

33. gonococcal endometritis, three months' duration _____

34. intestinal infection due to Campylobacter _____

35. shingles _____

Neoplasms

Using the Neoplasm Table in the Alphabetic Index, assign codes to the following diagnoses.

1. malignant primary neoplasm of the lower jawbone _____

2. benign neoplasm of the pharynx _____

3. neoplasm in situ, Wirsung's duct _____

4. neoplastic growth on the skin of the hip, uncertain behavior _____

5. secondary neoplasm on the posterior wall of the stomach _____

6. unspecified neoplasm of the pericardium _____

7. neoplasm of the mesopharynx, primary _____

8. cancer in situ, distal esophagus _____

9. benign tumor of the midbrain _____

10. spinal column neoplasm, primary _____

Using the Alphabetic Index and the Tabular List, provide codes for the following diagnoses.

11. secondary malignant neoplasm of the mediastinum _____

12. melanoma of the lip, malignant _____

13. Kaposi's sarcoma of the palate _____

14. benign neoplasm of the upper gum _____

15. dermatofibroma of skin of upper limb _____

16. malignant neoplasm of the testis _____

17. carcinoma in situ of the cervix uteri _____

18. malignant neoplasm of salivary gland, unspecified _____

19. malignant neoplasm of breast, upper-inner quadrant, female patient _____

20. neoplasm, ethmoid bone, malignant _____

21. neoplasm, malignant, upper lobe of lung _____

22. benign tumor of the rectosigmoid junction _____

23. carcinoma in situ, accessory sinuses _____

24. unspecified carcinoma of respiratory system _____

25. preinvasive carcinoma of the endometrium _____

26. subacute leukemia in remission _____

27. Hodgkin's granuloma, multiple lymph nodes _____

28. uterine fibromyoma _____

29. Letterer-Siwe disease, spleen _____

30. suspected primary carcinoma of the arm, screening test _____

31. ascites; possible carcinoma of the pancreas _____

32. cancer that has metastasized to the nose _____

33. cancer in situ of the temporal lobe _____

34. history of malignant neoplasm of stomach _____

35. screening mammogram, patient has family history of breast cancer and is considered high risk

    (*two codes*) _____

Endocrine, Nutritional, and Metabolic Diseases, and Immunity Disorders

Provide the codes for the following diagnoses.

1. congenital hypothyroidism _____

2. mucopolysaccharidosis _____

3. gouty arthropathy _____

4. macroglobulinemia _____

5. deficiency of vitamin K _____

6. medulloadrenal hyperfunction _____

7. kwashiorkor _____

8. Hashimoto's disease _____

9. Werner's syndrome _____

10. Lorain-Levi dwarfism _____

11. Fröhlich's syndrome _____

12. Pompe's disease _____

13. cystinuria _____

14. agammaglobulinemia, Bruton's type _____

15. dehydration _____

16. Nezelof's syndrome _____

17. acute thyroiditisv _____

18. dyshormonogenic goiter _____

19. Marie's syndrome _____

20. thyrocele _____

21. Harris' syndrome _____

22. mild malnutrition _____

23. pellagra _____

Note the fifth-digit subclassification requirement when assigning codes for the following diagnoses.

24. hypercalcemia _____

25. gouty tophi of ear _____

26. Grave's disease _____

27. diabetes mellitus, type I, uncontrolled _____

28. diabetes mellitus, type II _____

29. diabetes with ketoacidosis, adult-onset, controlled _____

30. insulin coma, patient with uncontrolled juvenile diabetes mellitus _____

31. diabetes with hypoglycemia, type I _____

32. uric acid nephrolithiasis _____

33. morbid obesity _____

34. Herrick's syndrome _____

35. obese patient encounter for dietary counseling (*two codes*) _____

Diseases of the Blood and Blood-Forming Organs

Provide the codes for the following diagnoses.

1. chlorotic anemia _____

2. anemia due to dietary deficiency of vitamin B 12 _____

3. sickle-cell anemia _____

4. hemophilia _____

5. hereditary hemolytic anemia _____

6. hereditary hemolytic anemia due to enzyme deficiency _____

7. stomatocytosis _____

8. specified hereditary hemolytic anemia not elsewhere classified _____

9. congenital elliptocytosis _____

10. iron deficiency anemia _____

11. Henoch's purpura _____

12. aplastic anemia due to chronic systemic disease _____

13. von Willebrand's disease _____

14. thrombocytopenia _____

15. secondary thrombocytopenia _____

16. sideroblastic anemia _____

17. congenital dyserythropoietic anemia _____

18. anemia _____

19. type II congenital nonspherocytic anemia _____

20. Runeberg's disease _____

Mental Disorders

Provide the codes for the following diagnoses.

1. mild mental retardation _____

2. depression _____

3. frontal lobe syndrome _____

4. tobacco dependence _____

5. subacute delirium _____

6. nonalcoholic Korsakoff's psychosis _____

7. neurotic anxiety disorder _____

8. depression with anxiety _____

9. panic attack _____

10. narcissistic personality disorder _____

Note the fifth-digit subclassification requirement when assigning codes for the following diagnoses.

11. continuous dependence on methadone _____

12. episodic cocaine abuse _____

13. mild tantrums _____

14. active disintegrative psychosis _____

15. severe mixed manic-depressive psychosis _____

16. chronic catatonic type schizophrenic disorder _____

17. single episode of manic disorder _____

18. occasional amphetamine abuse _____

19. drunkenness _____

20. dependence on barbiturates and morphine _____

Diseases of the Nervous System and Sense Organs

Hint: Some conditions require the assignment of two codes, one for the disease's etiology (origin or cause) and a second for its manifestation, or typical signs or symptoms. (On occasion, there is a single combination code for the etiology and the manifestation.) In the Alphabetic Index, a requirement for two codes is indicated when two codes appear after a term, the second of which is in brackets and italics. Likewise, the instruction "code first underlying disease" in the Tabular List indicates the need for two codes. (The alternative phrases "code first associated disorder" or "code first underlying disorder" may also be used.) The instruction appears below a code printed in italics. Codes shown in italics are never primary. These codes are for the *manifestation* only, not for the etiology, even when the diagnostic statement is written in that order.

Provide the codes for the following diagnoses.

1. Huntington's chorea _____
2. hereditary spastic paraplegia _____
3. paralysis _____
4. brachial plexus lesions _____
5. benign intracranial hypertension _____
6. blind hypotensive eye _____
7. cortical senile cataract _____
8. diplopia _____
9. visual field defect _____
10. achromatopsia _____
11. corneal ectasia _____
12. conjunctival xerosis _____
13. sensory disorder affecting eyelid function _____
14. stenosis of lacrimal sac _____
15. acute serous otitis media _____
16. wax in ear _____
17. acute tympanitis _____
18. aural vertigo _____
19. subjective tinnitus _____

20. central hearing loss _____

21. paralytic ptosis _____

22. mucopurulent conjunctivitis _____

23. primary open angle glaucoma _____

24. detached retina _____

For the following descriptions, provide both the etiology and manifestation codes in the correct order.
Hint: Remember to check for fifth-digit subclassification requirements.

25. meningitis in typhoid fever _____

26. toxic encephalitis due to exposure to mercury _____

27. childhood cerebral degeneration due to Hunter's disease _____

28. peripheral autonomic neuropathy in type II controlled diabetes _____

29. Eaton-Lambert syndrome due to pernicious anemia _____

30. myopathy from Addison's disease _____

31. retinal dystrophy in Fabry's disease _____

32. glaucoma in/with neurofibromatosis _____

33. diabetic cataract _____

34. exophthalmic ophthalmoplegia due to toxic diffuse goiter _____

35. chronic mycotic otitis externa because of otomycosis _____

Diseases of the Circulatory System

Provide the codes for the following diagnoses.

1. acute rhematic endocarditis _____
2. chronic rheumatic pericarditis _____
3. angina pectoris _____
4. preinfarction angina _____
5. chronic myocardial ischemia _____
6. chronic primary pulmonary hypertension _____
7. acute endocarditis _____
8. constrictive pericarditis _____
9. aortic valve stenosis _____
10. cardiomegaly _____
11. complete atrioventricular block _____
12. Moyamoya disease _____
13. intracerebral hemorrhage _____
14. postphlebitic syndrome without complication _____
15. Sydenham's chorea _____
16. tricuspid valve obstruction _____
17. old myocardial infarction _____
18. aneurysm of coronary vessels _____
19. arteriovenous fistula of pulmonary vessels _____
20. soldiers' patches _____
21. bleeding esophageal varicose veins _____
22. Wallgren's disease _____
23. blue phlebitis _____
24. atherosclerosis of extremties with intermittent claudication _____
25. stenocardia _____
26. heart failure following cardiac surgery _____
27. meningococcal infective endocarditis _____
28. Spens' syndrome _____

Be alert for fifth-digit subclassification requirements when assigning codes for the following diagnoses.

29. acute myocardial infarction _____

30. initial care of acute myocardial infarction of anterolateral wall _____

31. occlusion of basilar artery with cerebral infarction _____

32. cerebral thrombosis _____

33. stenosis of vertebral artery _____

34. Beck's syndrome _____

35. sinus tachycardia _____

Hint: Use the Hypertension Table in the Alphabetic Index to point to the various types of hypertensive disease. There are three subcategories of essential hypertension: malignant (401.0), benign (401.1), and unspecified (401.9). If the diagnostic statement does not contain the word *malignant* or *benign*, the hypertension is coded as unspecified. Hypertension may also be a coexisting condition; if so, two codes must be assigned, one for the primary condition and one for the hypertension, which is secondary in this case.

Using the Hypertension Table in the Alphabetic Index, assign codes to the following diagnoses.

36. benign hypertension due to brain tumor _____

37. unspecified hypertension due to renal artery stenosis _____

38. secondary malignant hypertension due to Cushing's disease _____

39. accelerated hypertension _____

40. intermittant vascular hypertensive disease _____

Some of the following diagnoses require two codes.

41. rheumatic aortic insufficiency and congestive heart failure _____

42. mitral and aortic valve insufficiency and atrial flutter _____

43. acute pericarditis caused by uremia _____

44. heart failure due to benign hypertension _____

45. hypertrophy of the heart due to malignant hypertension _____

46. cardiomyopathy due to excessive alcohol consumption _____

47. angina decubitus and essential hypertension _____

48. tuberculosis and endocarditis (unspecified) _____

49. peripheral angiopathy due to diabetes mellitus _____

50. inflammed varicose veins on the leg _____

Diseases of the Respiratory System

Provide the codes for the following diagnoses.

1. bronchiectasis without acute exacerbation _____
2. adenoid vegetations _____
3. deviated nasal septum _____
4. cellulitis of vocal cords _____
5. nasopharyngeal polyp _____
6. peritonsillar abscess _____
7. asbestosis _____
8. lung abscess _____
9. allergic bronchopulmonary aspergillosis _____
10. mediastinitis _____
11. idiopathic fibrosing alveolitis _____
12. asthma with acute exacerbation _____
13. pneumococcal pneumonia _____
14. allergic rhinitis due to pollen _____
15. chronic pulmonary congestion _____
16. acute nasopharyngitis _____
17. tracheal abscess _____
18. bronchitis _____
19. mucopurulent chronic bronchitis _____
20. acute and chronic obstructive bronchitis _____
21. chronic laryngitis _____
22. acute infective tonsillitis _____
23. acute bronchiolitis with bronchospasm _____
24. chronic maxillary sinus infection _____
25. extrinsic asthma with status asthmaticus _____

Some of the following diagnoses require two codes.

26. pneumonia in cytomegalic inclusion disease _____

27. pneumonia due to Pseudomonas _____

28. acute and chronic respiratory failure _____

29. adenoviral pneumonia and allergic bronchitis _____

30. asthma with chronic obstructive pulmonary disease _____

31. acute bronchitis with chronic obstructive pulmonary disease _____

32. acute pulmonary manifestations due to radiation _____

33. hypertrophy of nasal turbinates _____

34. hyperplasia of tonsils with adenoids _____

35. acute bronchiolitis due to RSV _____

Diseases of the Digestive System

Hint: Some conditions in the ICD-9-CM are classified with combination codes that cover both the illness, such as gastric or peptic ulcers, and a commonly associated condition, such as hemorrhage (bleeding) and/or perforation. Check carefully during the coding process to verify whether a combination code classifies both the etiology and the manifestation of the documented diagnosis.

Provide the codes for the following diagnoses.

1. anal abscess _____
2. appendicitis _____
3. reflux esophagitis _____
4. alveolitis of the jaw _____
5. acute gingivitis _____
6. arthralgia of temporomandibular joint _____
7. anodontia _____
8. glossodynia _____
9. sialoadenitis _____
10. perforated esophagus _____
11. hiatal hernia _____
12. gastric diverticulum _____
13. peritoneal adhesions following surgery _____
14. constipation (unspecified) _____
15. intestinal abscess _____
16. peritonitis _____
17. chronic persistent hepatitis _____
18. calculus of gallbladder with acute cholecystitis _____
19. acute cholecystitis _____
20. Crohn's disease _____
21. gangrenous umbilical hernia _____
22. acute gastritis with hemorrhage _____
23. acute perforated gastric ulcer _____

24. chronic obstructed gastric ulcer _____

25. perforated peptic ulcer _____

26. segmental ileitis _____

27. fecal impaction _____

28. cholestatic cirrhosis _____

Some of the following diagnoses require two codes.

29. hepatitis in mumps _____

30. hepatitis in Coxsackie virus disease _____

31. gastrojejunal ulcer with obstruction, hemorrhage, and perforation _____

32. strawberry gallbladder _____

33. acute and chronic cholecystitis _____

34. recurrent bilateral inguinal hernia _____

35. liver damage because of chronic alcoholism _____

Diseases of the Genitourinary System

Hint: If a code is followed in the Tabular List by the instruction "use additional code" or "code also" (or another phrase meaning the same thing), two codes are required. In some cases, the additional code classifies an associated condition or organism. If the underlying disease must be coded first, the instruction is "Code first". . ., and code order is the same as shown in the Alphabetic Index—etiology followed by manifestation.

Provide the codes for the following diagnoses.

1. renal failure _____

2. ureteric stone _____

3. mobile kidney _____

4. chronic interstitial cystitis _____

5. abscess of urethral gland _____

6. male infertility _____

7. galactocele _____

8. acute salpingitis and oophoritis _____

9. uterine endometriosis _____

10. ovarian cyst _____

11. cervical anaplasia _____

12. dysmenorrhea _____

13. fibrocystic breast disease _____

14. bladder paralysis _____

15. urethral diverticulum _____

16. female stress incontinence _____

17. hematuria _____

18. hydrocele male _____

19. stricture of vas deferens _____

20. spermatocele _____

21. acute glomerulonephritis

22. nephrosis _____

23. nonfunctioning gallbladder _____

24. renal disease _____

25. chocolate cyst _____

Provide two codes for each of the following diagnostic statements. Remember to check for fifth-digit subclassification requirements and to list codes in the correct order, if it is specified.

26. uremic pericarditis _____

27. enlarged prostate with urge and stress incontinence _____

28. prostatitis in blastomycosis _____

29. vaginitis due to Staphylococcus _____

30. female infertility due to postoperative peritubal adhesions _____

31. acute cystitis due to Escherichia coli organism _____

32. nephritis due to diabetes mellitus _____

33. pyelonenephritis due to renal tuberculosis _____

34. acute prostatitis due to Streptococcus _____

35. vulvovaginal gland abscess and female stress incontinence _____

Complications of Pregnancy, Childbirth, and the Puerperium

Provide codes for the following diagnoses.

1. hydatidiform mole _____

2. abdominal pregnancy without intrauterine pregnancy _____

3. complete spontaneous abortion complicated by renal failure _____

4. incomplete spontaneous abortion with complications _____

5. legally induced abortion _____

6. complete abortion complicated by shock _____

7. abortion _____

8. hemorrhage in early pregnancy _____

9. premature separation of placenta _____

10. mild hyperemesis gravidarum _____

11. antepartum hemorrhage _____

12. false labor _____

13. prolonged labor _____

14. post-term pregnancy, 41 weeks _____

15. essential hypertension complicating care _____

16. prenatal gestational proteinuria _____

17. rubella during pregnancy _____

18. gestational diabetes _____

19. eclamptic toxemia _____

20. delivery of triplets _____

21. uterine death of delivered late-term fetus _____

22. prolonged second stage labor _____

23. vulval hematoma after delivery _____

24. postpartum varicose veins in legs _____

25. antepartum deep-vein thrombosis _____

26. Rh incompatibility _____

27. delivery complicated by short umbilical cord _____

28. puerperal pulmonary embolism _____

29. nipple fissure in fourth week after childbirth _____

30. delivery complicated by inverted uterus _____

31. postpartum fibrinolysis _____

Provide two codes for each of the following diagnostic statements. Remember to check for fifth-digit subclassification requirements and to list codes in the correct order, if it is specified.

32. normal delivery of single liveborn _____

33. normal delivery of liveborn twins _____

34. normal delivery of quadruplets, three liveborn and one stillborn _____

35. delivery complicated by obstructed labor caused by face presentation _____

Diseases of the Skin and Subcutaneous Tissue

Provide codes for the following diagnoses.

1. allergic urticaria _____
2. sebaceous cyst _____
3. hirsutism _____
4. ingrowing nail _____
5. acquired keratoderma _____
6. clavus _____
7. lichenification _____
8. parapsoriasis _____
9. Ritter's disease _____
10. dermatosis herpetiformis _____
11. dermatitis vegetans _____
12. diaper rash _____
13. contact dermatitis due to detergents _____
14. dermatitis due to furs _____
15. Sneddon-Wilkinson syndrome _____
16. ocular pemphigus _____
17. Lyell's syndrome _____
18. chronic parapsoriasis lichenoides _____
19. localized dermatosclerosis _____
20. Koilonychia _____
21. Hebra's prurigo _____
22. striata lichen _____
23. lupoid sycosis _____
24. comedo _____
25. chronic ulcer of neck _____
26. DSAP (disseminated superficial actinic porokeratosis) _____
27. herald patch _____
28. paronychia of big toe _____
29. psoriatic arthropathy _____

Provide two codes for each of the following diagnostic statements. Remember to check for fifth-digit subclassification requirements and to list codes in the correct order, if it is specified.

30. winter itch and prurigo nodularis _____

31. photoallergic response due to uric acid metabolism drug _____

32. abscess of cheek due to Staphylococcus aureus _____

33. seborrhea and pustular acne _____

34. prickly heat rash and hidradenitis suppurative _____

35. boils on wrist and shoulder _____

Diseases of the Musculoskeletal System and Connective Tissue

Provide the codes for the following diseases.

1. hallux varus, right great toe _____

2. senile osteoporosis _____

3. bunion _____

4. limb pain _____

5. pain in lower back _____

6. cervicalgia _____

7. Schmorl's nodes of the lumbar region _____

8. calcaneal spur _____

9. patellar chondromalacia _____

10. systemic sclerosis _____

11. rheumatoid carditis _____

12. collagen disease _____

13. primary generalized osteoarthrosis, multiple sites _____

14. allergic arthritis _____

15. acute osteomyelitis of the lower leg _____

16. periostitis of shoulder _____

17. Baker's cyst _____

18. myofibrosis _____

19. chronic osteomyelitis _____

20. unicameral bone cyst _____

21. malunion of fracture _____

22. acquired clubfoot _____

23. postural lordosis _____

24. acquired talipes planus _____

25. thoracogenic scoliosis _____

26. old rupture of meniscus of scapula _____

27. metatarsal arthralgia _____

28. Paget's bone disease _____

29. aseptic necrosis of medial femoral condyle _____

30. Legg-Calvé-Perthes disease _____

Provide two codes for each of the following diagnostic statements. Remember to check for fourth- and fifth-digit requirements and to list codes in the correct order, if it is specified.

31. upper arm arthropathy in Behcet's syndrome _____

32. arthropathic knee associated with ulcerative enterocolitis _____

33. vertebral column osteopathy due to infantile paralytic poliomyelitis _____

34. chronic osteomyelitis of glenohumeral joint and elbow joint _____

35. ruptured extensor and flexor tendons, hand _____

Congenital Anomalies

Provide codes for the following diagnoses.

1. congenital absence of vertebra _____

2. unilateral congenital hip dislocation _____

3. exstrophy of urinary bladder _____

4. undescended testis _____

5. congenital cystic liver disease _____

6. Hirschsprung's disease _____

7. aglossia _____

8. web of larynx _____

9. Scimitar syndrome _____

10. posterior atresia of nares _____

11. cleft palate with cleft lip _____

12. congenital laryngeal stenosis _____

13. pancreatic hypoplasia _____

14. autosomal dominant polycystic kidney _____

15. congenital atresia of the urethra _____

16. multiple symphalangy _____

17. deformity of clavicle, congenital _____

18. prune belly syndrome _____

19. translocation Down's syndrome _____

20. hereditary trophedema _____

Conditions Originating in the Perinatal Period

Provide codes for the following diagnoses.

1. prematurity _____

2. fetal alcohol syndrome _____

3. fetus affected by the mother's malnutrition _____

4. neonatal hepatitis _____

5. respiratory distress syndrome _____

6. hyperthermia in newborn _____

7. anemia of prematurity _____

8. convulsions in newborn _____

9. neonatal superficial hematoma _____

10. congenital rubella _____

11. wet lung syndrome _____

12. neonatal Candida infection _____

13. anemia due to RH isoimmunization _____

14. moderate birth asphyxia _____

15. acute neonatal hydramnios _____

Provide a V code and a code from the range 760–779 for the following diagnoses.

16. hospital birth of living child, infant is premature and weighs 2000 grams

    _____

17. hospital birth of twin, mate liveborn, neonatal pulmonary immaturity

    _____

18. full-term birth in hospital of living male child, delivered by cesarean section, with neonatal transient hyperthyroidism _____

19. post-term birth in hospital of twin, mate stillborn _____

20. premature birth of female twins, first child delivered in ambulance en route to hospital, second child delivered in hospital _____

Symptoms, Signs, and Ill-Defined Conditions

Provide codes for the following diagnoses.

1. coma _____

2. fainting _____

3. abnormal electrocardiogram _____

4. viremia _____

5. abnormal blood glucose tolerance test _____

6. splenomegaly _____

7. urge incontinence _____

8. wheezing _____

9. hiccough _____

10. fever _____

11. hypersomnia with sleep apnea _____

12. chronic fatigue syndrome _____

13. carpopedal spasm _____

14. cyanosis _____

15. renal colic _____

16. head pain _____

17. palpitations _____

18. hypernasality when speaking _____

19. short stature in childhood _____

20. staggering when walking _____

21. Dupré's syndrome _____

22. finding of nonspecific serologic evidence of HIV _____

23. finding of abnormal basal metabolic rate _____

24. abdominal cramping _____

25. generalized rigidity of the abdomen _____

26. ascites in the lower left quadrant of the abdomen _____

27. mass in epigastric area of abdomen _____

28. exanthem _____

29. nausea with vomiting _____

30. nosebleed _____

Provide two codes for each of the following diagnostic statements. Remember to check for fourth- and fifth-digit requirements and to list codes in the correct order, if it is specified.

31. elevated blood pressure and nervousness _____

32. pallor and flushing _____

33. gangrene due to diabetes _____

34. continuous urinary incontinence because of complete uterovaginal prolapse

_____

35. precordial pain and hyperventilation _____

Injury and Poisoning

Provide codes for the following diagnoses.

1. open fracture of nasal bones _____

2. closed fracture of sacrum and coccyx _____

3. open fracture of lumbar with spinal cord injury _____

4. closed fracture of big toe _____

5. metacarpophalangeal joint sprain _____

6. strained sacroiliac ligament _____

7. concussion with moderate loss of consciousness _____

8. internal laceration to lung with open wound into thorax _____

9. ocular laceration _____

10. open wound of nasal septum _____

11. complicated wound of upper arm _____

12. esophageal bruise _____

13. black eye _____

14. swallowed foreign body _____

15. injury to auditory nerve _____

16. immediate shock after an injury _____

17. hematoma of heel _____

18. animal bite on knee _____

19. rupture of rotator cuff (traumatic) _____

20. left ear avulsion _____

21. closed posterior humeral dislocation _____

22. closed Dupuytren's fracture _____

23. closed fracture of the acromial process _____

24. fractured wrist _____

25. greenstick fracture, condylar process, mandible _____

26. open fracture of base of skull, with cerebral laceration, contusion, and concussion _____

27. ruptured superior vena cava _____

28. closed fracture of cervical vertebra with spinal nerve injury, C1–C4 _____

29. fracture of distal phalanges _____

30. pneumohemothorax _____

Provide an injury code and an E code for each of the following diagnostic statements.

31. 7 ribs fractured due to fall from forklift truck _____

32. lacerations to hand from broken glass _____

33. forearm crushed under packing crate _____

34. bruise on buttock from fall during a horseback ride _____

35. snow blower accident caused multiple open wounds of lower limb _____

Provide two codes for each of the following burns.

36. third-degree burns of face, head, and neck *Hint:* Provide a code for the burn degree and location, and a code for the 9% TBSA third-degree burn. _____

37. first-degree burn of thigh, lower leg, and foot _____

38. blistered palms _____

39. full-thickness skin loss of front and back of trunk _____

40. third-degree burns of both legs and back _____

Identify the codes for the following substances in the Table of Drugs and Chemicals.

41. carbitol _____

42. calomel _____

43. iron compounds _____

44. soluble hexobarbitone _____

45. hornet sting _____

Provide codes for the following diagnoses.

46. tick paralysis _____

47. ampicillin taken in error _____

48. overdose of Levodopa _____

49. toxic effect of petroleum products _____

50. Minamata disease _____

51. toxic effect of rubbing alcohol _____

52. toxic effect, fumes of lead salts _____

53. heat cramps _____

54. accidental hypothermia _____

55. heat prostration _____

56. toxic effect of lye _____

57. poisoning by topical dental drugs _____

58. poisoning from local anesthetic _____

59. poisoning by psychotropic agent _____

60. methadone poisoning _____

61. overdose of ovarian hormones _____

62. poisoning by coronary vasodilator _____

63. Coumarin poisoning _____

64. radiation sickness _____

65. anaphylactic shock after eating peanuts _____

For the following late effects of injuries, provide two codes in the correct order.

66. nausea as a late effect of radiation sickness _____

67. pain from an old fractured shoulder blade _____

68. swelling due to old contusion of knee _____

69. abdominal mass due to a previous spleen injury _____

70. abnormal posture due to old sciatic nerve injury _____

Practice Using CPT

1. For each term, underline the word that you would look for in the index of CPT.

    A. Intracapsular lens extraction

    B. Coombs test

    C. X-ray of duodenum

    D. Unlisted procedure, maxillofacial prosthetics

    E. DTAP immunization

2. Identify the symbol used to indicate a new procedure code, and list five new codes that appear in CPT.

    _____

    _____

    _____

    _____

    _____

    _____

3. Identify the symbol used to indicate a procedure that is usually done in addition to a primary procedure. Locate code 92981, and describe the unit of measure that is involved with this add-on code.

    _____

    _____

    _____

    _____

    _____

    _____

4. Identify the symbol that indicates that the code's description has been changed, and list five examples of codes with new or revised descriptors that appear in CPT.

    _____

    _____

    _____

    _____

    _____

    _____

5. Identify the symbols that enclose new or revised text other than the code's descriptor, and list five examples of codes with new or revised text that appear in CPT.

_____

_____

_____

_____

_____

_____

Modifiers

Provide the correct modifier for each of the following descriptions.

1. multiple modifiers _____

2. distinct procedural service _____

3. prolonged Evaluation and Management service _____

4. staged procedure _____

5. assistant surgeon _____

6. discontinued procedure _____

7. repeat procedure by same physician _____

8. unusual anesthesia _____

9. mandated services _____

10. surgical team _____

11. physician provides follow-up care after another physician has performed surgery _____

12. puncture aspiration of a cyst in each breast _____

13. radiologist provides a report on a lateral chest X ray _____

14. surgery was discontinued because the patient went into shock during the operation

    _____

15. surgeon administers a regional Bier block _____

16. patient hemorrhaged heavily during surgery; procedure took twice as long as typically required to

    perform _____

17. surgeon repairs the flexor tendon of the foot and excises a ganglion on the fourth toe

    _____

18. during an operation, a thoracic surgeon provides surgical access to the spine while an orthopedist

    performs a spinal fusion _____

19. surgeon provides part of a procedure _____

20. patient is returned to the operating room three hours after surgery because of ruptured sutures

    _____

Evaluation and Management

Section A

1. In which category—problem-focused, expanded problem-focused, detailed, or comprehensive—would you place these statements concerning patient history? Why?

   Case A Patient seen for follow-up of persistent sinus problems including pain, stuffiness, and greenish drainage over the past twenty days. She continues to have left-sided pain in the forehead and maxillary areas and feels that her symptoms are worse around dust. She gets drainage into her throat, which causes her to cough. Review of systems reveals no history of diabetes or asthma. She has thyroid problems for which she takes Synthroid®.

   Category _____

   _____

   Case B Patient presents with a mild case of poison ivy on face and both hands contracted four days ago while gardening; has never been bothered by poison ivy before.

   Category _____

   _____

2. Using the office visit E/M codes, which code would you select for each of these cases?

   Case A Chart note for established patient:
   S: Patient returns for removal of stitches I placed about seven days ago. Reports normal itching around the wound area, but no pain or swelling.
   O: Wound at lateral aspect of the left eye looks well healed. Decision made to remove the 5-0 nylon sutures, which was done without difficulty.
   A: Laceration, healed.
   P: Patient advised to use vitamin E for scar prophylaxis.

   E/M Code _____

   Case B Initial office evaluation by oncologist of a sixty-five-year-old female with sudden unexplained twenty-pound weight loss. Comprehensive history and examination performed.

   E/M Code _____

   Case C Office visit by established patient for regularly scheduled blood test to monitor long-term effects of Coumadin; nurse spends five minutes, reviews the test, confirms that the patient is feeling well, and states that no change in the dosage is necessary.

   E/M Code _____

Section B

Provide procedure codes from the Evaluation and Management Section for the following procedures.

1. initial office visit, 25-year-old male, with boil on back; physician took a brief history, performed a limited examination of the back, and there were little risk of complications and minimal treatment options _____

2. office visit, established patient is a 67-year-old female, with controlled diabetes mellitus, complaining of lack of sensation in her feet; expanded problem-focused history and examination _____

3. first hospital visit, admitting physician, comprehensive history, examination, and moderate decision making _____

4. initial office consultation; detailed history and examination, low complexity medical decision making _____

5. annual comprehensive physical examination for 11-year-old new patient _____

6. medical disability examination by physician employed by state _____

7. hospital visit to previously admitted patient; problem-focused history and examination, 10 minutes spent at bedside _____

8. emergency department service for patient following a car accident; comprehensive history and examination, highly complex decision making _____

9. discharge of patient from nursing home, 45 minute encounter _____

10. home visit for established patient, straightforward case, problem-focused examination _____

11. first visit to provide consultation on hospitalized patient, minor problems, brief visit _____

12. direction of EMS care _____

13. one hour of critical care _____

14. subsequent care of critically ill and unstable infant, 25 days old, in intensive care _____

15. subsequent care for new patient in a long-term care facility; patient regaining movement and has an excellent prognosis _____

16. supervision of hospice patient care (25 minutes spent in one month) _____

17. 55-minute medical conference, with other health care providers, related to the patient's overall care _____

18. one-hour physician attendance as standby during delivery; mother has uncontrolled diabetes mellitus _____

19. brief telephone call by physician to patient _____

20. 75 minutes of group counseling for risk-factor reduction _____

21. newborn care provided in parents' home _____

In addition to E/M codes, provide modifiers and additional procedure codes if appropriate for the following.

22. comprehensive annual examination for established 65-year-old patient

    _____

23. primary care physician sends a patient to a cardiologist for an evaluation of a complicated vascular problem; during the hour-long encounter, the specialist performs a comprehensive history and examination, and follows up the visit with a written report to the PCP; MDM was moderate

    _____

24. thoracic surgeon provides a second opinion on the appropriateness of a single bypass procedure as requested by a third-party payer; a detailed history and examination are obtained; MDM is of low complexity _____

25. during an annual physical examination, a 45-year-old established patient complains of general tiredness and severe shortness of breath during mild activity; physician performs a detailed cardiovascular assessment with additional detailed history; following complex MDM, the physician also schedules an immediate complete heart study _____

CPT Review; Anesthesia Section

Section A

Match the key terms with the correct definitions.

   A. panel
   B. professional component
   C. separate procedure
   D. Category III codes
   E. global period
   F. bundled code
   G. Category II codes
   H. add-on code
   I. unlisted procedure
   J. modifier

_____ 1. The physician's skill, time, and expertise used in performing a procedure

_____ 2. Temporary codes for emerging technology, services, and procedures

_____ 3. Procedure code that groups related procedures under a single code

_____ 4. A service that is not listed in CPT and requires a special report

_____ 5. The inclusion of postoperative care for a specified period in the charges for a surgical procedure

_____ 6. CPT codes that are used to track performance measurement

_____ 7. In CPT, a single code that groups laboratory tests that are frequently done together

_____ 8. A procedure performed in addition to a primary procedure

_____ 9. A secondary procedure that is performed with a primary procedure and that is indicated in CPT by a plus sign (+) next to the code

_____10. A two-digit number indicating that special circumstances were involved with a procedure, such as a reduced service or a discontinued procedure

Section B

Provide the CPT code for each of the following anesthesia services. *Hint:* All codes are in the Anesthesia Section.

1. cesarean delivery _____

2. arthroscopic procedures of the hip joint _____

3. transurethral resection of prostate _____

4. breast reconstruction _____

5. heart transplant _____

6. needle biopsy of thyroid _____

7. repair of cleft palate _____

8. cervical spine procedure _____

9. esophageal procedure _____

10. thoracoplasty _____

11. radical hysterectomy _____

12. chemonucleolysis _____

13. Whipple procedure, upper abdomen _____

14. bilateral orchiopexy _____

15. hysterosalpingography _____

16. embolectomy of the femoral artery _____

17. closed ulnar procedure _____

18. Strayer procedure _____

19. arthroscopic procedure, shoulder joint _____

20. repair of shoulder cast _____

21. needle arteriogram of carotid artery _____

22. continuous epidural, labor and vaginal delivery _____

Provide the anesthesia code and a modifier for the following services.

23. procedure on popliteal bursa, patient with mild systemic disease _____

24. open procedure, sacroiliac joint, normal patient _____

25. major abdominal vessel procedure for patient with life-threatening disease

_____

26. plastic repair, cleft lip, six-month old _____

27. amniocentesis, healthy mother _____

28. spinal fluid shunting procedure on moribund patient _____

29. anesthesia is induced but blepharoplasty is canceled _____

30. amputation, ankle and foot, severely diabetic patient _____

31. emergency-room appendectomy _____

32. arthroscopic procedure of knee joint, mildly arthritic patient _____

33. cardiac catheterization for patient with malignant hypertension _____

34. removal of donated organs from brain-dead patient _____

35. pneumocentesis, elderly patient _____

Surgery: Integumentary System

Provide the integumentary system codes for the following procedures.

1. simple incision and removal of foreign body from subcutaneous tissue _____

2. complicated I & D, abscess _____

3. excision of benign lesion, 0.5 cm diameter, from the upper arm _____

4. excision of a 2.1 cm benign lesion from the foot _____

5. abrasion of a single lesion _____

6. cervicoplasty _____

7. rhytidectomy of glabellar frown lines _____

8. escharotomy _____

9. breast reduction _____

10. breast reconstruction with free flap _____

11. lumpectomy _____

12. lactiferous duct fistula, excision _____

13. destruction of a malignant lesion, 4.1 cm, on nose _____

14. chemical exfoliation for acne _____

15. initial local treatment for first-degree burn _____

16. punch graft for hair transplant, 12 punch grafts _____

17. shaving of a dermal lesion on the scalp, 1.4 cm, local anesthesia _____

18. nine injections into a lesion _____

19. repair of nail bed _____

20. neurovascular pedicle flap _____

21. facial epidermal chemical peel _____

Some of the following procedures require two codes and/or the use of a modifier.

22. excision and simple closure of 3.3 cm malignant lesion on upper leg

    _____

23. extremely complicated excision of benign congenital cyst, 2.5 cm, on chest, requiring twice the expected time in surgery _____

24. excision of a 0.3 cm benign lesion on each ear _____

25. implanting contraceptive capsules _____

26. excision of malignant lesions, 1.1 cm on upper arm and 0.1 cm on foot

    _____

27. split graft, 80 sq cm, lower leg, staged procedure on infant

    _____

28. surgical removal of excess skin and tissue from upper arm and hand

    _____

29. needle core biopsy of both breasts not using imaging guidance

    _____

30. preparation and insertion of custom breast implant five days after mastectomy

    _____

Hint: Each of the following procedures requires add-on codes.

31. abrasion, nine lesions _____

32. application of 200 sq cm skin xenograft _____

33. laser destruction of four premalignant lesions _____

34. debridement of infected skin, 18 percent of body surface _____

35. complex repair of wound on trunk, 12 cm _____

Surgery: Musculoskeletal System

Provide the musculoskeletal system codes for the following procedures.

1. removal of body cast applied by another physician _____

2. primary repair of ruptured Achilles tendon _____

3. tendon sheath incision _____

4. closed treatment of fractured ulnar shaft _____

5. complete wrist arthrodesis _____

6. humeral osteotomy _____

7. closed treatment of sesamoid fracture _____

8. open treatment of talus fracture _____

9. I & D of foot bursa _____

10. elbow joint arthrodesisv _____

11. lateral fasciotomy with partial ostectomy _____

12. distal humeral sequestrectomy _____

13. repair of humeral nonunion with iliac graft _____

14. reinsertion of spinal fixation device _____

15. posterior arthrodesis for spinal deformity with cast _____

16. radial and ulnar osteotomy _____

17. amputation of tip of right thumb with direct closure _____

18. total hip replacement _____

19. percutaneous skeletal fixation of posterior pelvic ring dislocation _____

20. hip socket fracture, closed treatment, with manipulation and traction _____

21. trocar biopsy of rib _____

22. craterization of proximal humerus _____

23. anterior capsulorrhaphy, transfer of coracoid process _____

24. surgical removal of prepatellar bursa _____

25. low back replacement strapping _____

Some of the following procedures require two codes and/or the use of a modifier.

26. Keller procedure, left and right halluces _____

27. surgical exploration of chest wound with debridement and removal of foreign body

    _____

28. arthrodesis of sacroiliac joint, graft harvested _____

29. talectomy provided during global period of previous unrelated surgery

    _____

30. medial and lateral meniscectomy _____

31. closed treatment of ankle dislocation under anesthesia with percutaneous skeletal fixation

    _____

32. epiphyseal arrest of distal femur, proximal tibia, and proximal fibula

    _____

33. closed treatment of dislocated sternoclavicular joint and patella

    _____

34. synovial biopsy and diagnostic arthroscopy of hip _____

35. surgical arthroscopy, ankle, with removal of foreign body

    _____

Surgery: Respiratory System

Provide the respiratory system codes for the following procedures. Include any necessary modifiers.

1. maxillectomy _____

2. maxillary sinus irrigation _____

3. total laryngectomy _____

4. closed laryngeal fracture treatment _____

5. simple revision of tracheostoma _____

6. cervical tracheoplasty _____

7. parietal pleurectomy _____

8. extrapleural thoracoplasty _____

9. complex surgical removal of dermoid cyst from nose _____

10. lateral rhinotomy to remove object from nose _____

11. intranasal sinusotomy, both maxillary sinuses _____

12. thyrotomy for tumor removal _____

13. emergency intubation tube _____

14. thoracentesis and tube insertion _____

15. catheterization with bronchial brush biopsy _____

16. surgical removal of two lobes of the lung _____

17. turbinate reduction _____

18. primary complete rhinoplasty _____

19. sinus endoscopy with anterior/posterior ethmoidectomy _____

20. anterovertical hemilaryngectomy _____

21. diagnostic bronchoscopy _____

22. flexible bronchoscopy with destruction of tumor by laser _____

23. unusually complicated revision of tracheostomy scar _____

24. puncture of both lungs for aspiration _____

25. bilateral lung transplantation _____

Some of the following procedures require two codes. *Hint:* For endoscopic procedures, read the notes before this code group carefully.

26. surgical thoracoscopy with excisions of pericardial and mediastinal cysts

    _____

27. surgical nasal/sinus endoscopy with maxillary antrostomy _____

28. planned tracheostomy on infant _____

29. hematoma drainage from nasal septum _____

30. laser destruction of two intranasal lesions, internal approach _____

31. sinusotomy, three paranasal sinuses _____

32. bilateral nasal evaluation using endoscope _____

33. direct diagnostic laryngoscopy and tracheoscopy with operating microscope

    _____

34. diagnostic nasal/sinus endoscopy with sphenoid sinusoscopy and inspection of interior nasal cavity, spheno-ethmoid recess and turbinates _____

35. turbinate excision followed by intranasal antrotomy _____

Surgery: Cardiovascular System

Provide the cardiovascular system codes for the following procedures. Include any necessary modifiers.

1. removal of permanent pacemaker pulse generator _____

2. mitral valve valvotomy, closed heart _____

3. coronary artery bypass using single venous graft _____

4. myocardial resection _____

5. repair of complete atrioventricular canal _____

6. saphenopopliteal vein anastomosis _____

7. carotid thromboendarterectomy _____

8. exploration of femoral artery _____

9. intravenous introduction of intracatheter _____

10. closure of ventricular septal defect _____

11. temporary pacemaker insertion _____

12. insertion of implantable intra-arterial infusion pump _____

13. pericardiectomy with cardiopulmonary bypass _____

14. insertion of transvenous electrode for dual chamber pacing cardioverter-defibrillator; initial insertion done 20 days earlier _____

15. aortic suture repair _____

16. discontinued pulmonary valve replacement _____

17. repair of transposed great arteries by aortic pulmonary artery reconstruction

    _____

18. pulmonary artery embolectomy _____

19. pulmonary artery banding _____

20. sinus of Valsalva aneurysm repair with cardiopulmonary bypass _____

21. ligation of secondary varicose veins, left and right legs _____

22. pulmonary endarterectomy with cardiopulmonary bypass _____

23. repair by division of patent ductus ateriosus in 10-year-old _____

24. graft, descending thoracic aorta _____

25. ring insertion and valvuloplasty, tricuspid valve _____

The following procedures may require two codes and/or the use of modifiers.

26. subcutaneous removal of pacing cardioverter-defibrillator pulse generator, electrodes removed by thoracotomy _____

27. subsequent pericardiocentesis with radiological S&I

_____

28. revision of skin pocket for pacing cardioverter-defibrillator

_____

29. aortic valve replacement using a homograft valve with cardiopulmonary bypass

_____

30. coronary artery bypass with one arterial graft and three venous grafts

_____

31. carotid and axillary-axillary arterial bypass with venous grafts

_____

32. radiological S&I for percutaneous transluminal balloon angioplasty

_____

33. excision of infected abdominal graft, surgical care only

_____

34. central venous catheter placed percutaneously in adult

_____

35. routine venipuncture _____

Surgery: Hemic and Lymphatic Systems; Mediastinum and Diaphragm

Provide codes for the following procedures. Include any necessary modifiers. In some cases, more than one code is required.

1. extensive drainage of lymphadenitis _____

2. injection procedure for identification of sentinel node

    _____

3. laceration repair, diaphragm _____

4. mediastinoscopy _____

5. needle biopsy of lymph node _____

6. axillary excision of cystic hygroma _____

7. pelvic lymphadenectomy _____

8. laparoscopic splenectomy _____

9. total splenectomy _____

10. autologous stem cell transplantation _____

11. retroperitoneal limited lymphadenectomy for staging

    _____

12. injection for lymphangiography _____

13. repair of chronic traumatic diaphragmatic hernia _____

14. lymphangiotomy _____

15. repair of ruptured spleen with partial splenectomy _____

16. insertion of cannula in thoracic duct _____

17. mediastinotomy with removal of object via cervical approach

    _____

18. injection procedure for splenoportography with radiological S&I

    _____

19. complete axillary lymphadenectomy and regional thoracic lymphadenectomy

    _____

20. injection procedure for bilateral pelvic/abdominal lymphangiography with radiological S&I

    _____

Surgery: Digestive System

Provide codes for the following procedures. Include any necessary modifiers. In some cases, more than one code is required.

1. resection of 50 percent of lip _____

2. repair of sliding inguinal hernia _____

3. insertion of peritoneal-venous shunt _____

4. exploratory laparotomy _____

5. removal of pancreatic calculus _____

6. cholecystectomy _____

7. portoenterostomy _____

8. wedge biopsy of liver _____

9. excision of Meckel's diverticulum _____

10. gastroduodenostomy _____

11. esophagoplasty, cervical approach _____

12. diagnostic esophagoscopy _____

13. esophagoscopy with polyp removal by snare technique

   _____

14. simple secondary control of oropharyngeal hemorrhage

   _____

15. excision of tonsil tags _____

16. primary repair, salivary duct _____

17. hemiglossectomy _____

18. repair of left and right incarcerated recurrent femoral hernias

   _____

19. percutaneous drainage of pancreatic pseudocyst with radiological S&I

   _____

20. diagnostic laparoscopy (separate procedure) _____

21. laparoscopic jejunostomy _____

22. esophageal dilation with 35 mm balloon with radiological S&I

   _____

23. Nissen fundoplasty _____

24. upper gastrointestinal endoscopy from esophagus to the jejunum with multiple biopsies

 _____

25. removal of object from mouth vestibule, discontinued procedure

 _____

26. frenotomy _____

27. palate resection, repeated procedure by same physician

 _____

28. secondary adenoidectomy, 10-year-old patient _____

29. near total esophagectomy with pharyngogastrostomy (without thoracotomy)

 _____

30. percutaneous placement of gastrostomy tube with radiological S&I

 _____

31. endoscopic placement of gastrostomy tube with radiological S&I

 _____

32. simple ileostomy revision done during same operative session as pharangeal wound suture

 _____

33. partial colectomy with ileostomy and creation of mucofistula

 _____

34. excision of ruptured appendix _____

35. diagnostic and surgical flexible colonoscopy past the splenic flexure and tumor removal by bipolar cautery _____

Surgery: Urinary System

Provide codes for the following procedures. Include any necessary modifiers. In some cases, more than one code is required.

1. ureterotomy _____

2. ureteroplasty _____

3. ureteral endoscopy through established ureterostomy

   _____

4. first-stage urethroplasty _____

5. drainage, deep periurethral abscess _____

6. cystourethroscopy with double-J type stent _____

7. closure of cystostomy _____

8. EMG studies of urethral sphincter _____

9. trocar bladder aspiration _____

10. simple bladder irrigation _____

11. ureteroileal conduit and Bricker operation _____

12. lithotripsy _____

13. laparoscopic nephrectomy _____

14. recipient nephrectomy, both kidneys _____

15. percutaneous needle renal biopsy with radiological S&I (fluoroscopy)

    _____

16. bilateral cystourethroscopy with ureteral meatotomy

    _____

17. complicated Foley Y-pyeloplasty _____

18. renal endoscopy through nephrotomy _____

19. complete transurethral resection of prostate (electrosurgical)

    _____

20. completion (second stage) of transurethral prostate resection *Hint*: Include a modifier.

    _____

21. laparoscopic sling suspension _____

22. cystourethroscopy with fulguration of 3.0 cm bladder tumor

_____

23. unilateral ureteroneocystostomy and cystourethroplasty

_____

24. transurethral resection, obstructive tissue, 18 months after a TURP

_____

25. discontinued contact laser vaporization of prostate _____

Surgery: Male Genital System; Intersex Surgery

Provide codes for the following procedures. Include any necessary modifiers. In some cases, more than one code is required.

1. testicular injury repair _____

2. bilateral simple orchiectomy _____

3. bilateral vasectomy _____

4. complicated vesiculotomy _____

5. laparoscopic orchiopexy _____

6. radical perineal prostatectomy _____

7. excision of Mullerian duct cyst _____

8. ligation of vas deferens _____

9. removal of foreign body, scrotum _____

10. I&D, abscess of epididymis _____

11. fixation of contralateral testis _____

12. unrelated plastic operation of penis during global period

    _____

13. incisional biopsy of testis followed by radical orchiectomy for tumor, inguinal approach

    _____

14. simple electrodesiccation of four lesions on penis _____

15. surgical excision of papilloma on penis, extensive procedure

    _____

16. injection procedure and excision of penile plaque in Peyronie disease

    _____

17. spermatocele excision _____

18. incisional prostate biopsy _____

19. spermatic vein ligation for varicocele, discontinued service

    _____

20. spermatic vein ligation for varicocele, laparoscopic surgery

    _____

21. clamp circumcision of newborn _____

22. corpora cavernosography with radiological S&I _____

23. deep penile I&D _____

24. Cecil repair, third stage _____

25. repair, hypospadias cripple _____

Surgery: Female Genital System and Maternity Care/Delivery

Provide codes for the following procedures. Include any necessary modifiers. In some cases, more than one code is required.

1. simple destruction of four lesions, vulva _____

2. complete radical vulvectomy _____

3. fitting and insertion of pessary _____

4. laser destruction of vaginal lesions simple _____

5. D&C, cervical stump _____

6. D&C, postpartum hemorrhage _____

7. uterine suspension _____

8. total abdominal hysterectomy _____

9. subtotal hysterectomy _____

10. insertion of IUD _____

11. diagnostic hysteroscopy _____

12. intrauterine embryo transfer _____

13. bilateral drainage of ovarian cysts by abdominal approach
    _____

14. bilateral complete salpingo-oophorectomy _____

15. radical abdominal hysterectomy with salpingo-oophorectomy

    _____

16. intra-uterine artificial insemination, unrelated procedure

    _____

17. vulvular biopsy of five lesions _____

18. vaginectomy and complete removal of vaginal wall _____

19. routine obstetric care/vaginal delivery _____

20. five visits for antepartum care only _____

21. abdominal hysterotomy, surgery only _____

22. hysterotomy and tubal ligation _____

23. cordocentesis with radiological S&I _____

24. laparoscopic treatment of ectopic pregnancy with salpingo-oophorectomy

_____

25. delivery, placenta _____

26. routine obstetric care/vaginal delivery, patient had previous cesarean delivery

_____

27. miscarriage surgically completed in first trimester _____

28. abortion induced by D&C _____

29. cesarean delivery, surgical care only _____

30. cesarean delivery, including postpartum care, and total hysterectomy following attempted vaginal delivery; patient had previous cesarean delivery _____

31. Strassman type hysteroplasty and closure of vesicouterine fistula

_____

32. chromotubation of oviduct including materials _____

33. laparoscopic assisted vaginal hysterectomy (uterus less than 250 grams)

_____

34. multifetal pregnancy reductions _____

35. episiotomy by assisting physician _____

Surgery: Endocrine System and Nervous System

Provide codes for the following procedures. Include any necessary modifiers. In some cases, more than one code is required.

1. total thyroid lobectomy _____

2. twist drill hole for subdural puncture _____

3. resection of a vascular lesion at the base of the posterior cranial fossa

    _____

4. craniotomy for repair of dural/CSF leak _____

5. exploratory craniectomy _____

6. aspiration of thyroid cyst _____

7. laparoscopic adrenalectomy _____

8. parathyroidectomy _____

9. total thyroidectomy, limited neck dissection, for excision of malignancy

    _____

10. adrenalectomy _____

11. subsequent subdural tap through suture, infant _____

12. subtemporal cranial decompression _____

13. craniotomy with elevation of bone flap for total hemispherectomy

    _____

14. craniotomy with frontal bone flap for craniosynostosis

    _____

15. obliteration of carotid aneurysm by dissection _____

16. removal of intracranial neurostimulator electrodes

    _____

17. creation of ventricular peritoneal CSF shunt _____

18. needle biopsy of spinal cord, with supervision and interpretation of computerized tomography

    guidance _____

19. implantation of intrathecal drug infusion programmable pump

    _____

20. lumbar laminectomy with exploration and decompression

_____

21. epidural percutaneous implantation of neurostimulator electrodes

_____

22. implantation of cranial nerve neurostimulator electrodes

_____

Provide codes and decide whether to append the -51 modifier.

23. craniectomy, infratentorial, to excise a brain abscess, and twist drill hole to implant ventricular catheter _____

24. craniectomy, supratentorial and infratentorial, for drainage of intracranial abscess

_____

25. vertebral corpectomy with decompression of spinal cord, three segments

_____

Surgery: Eye and Ocular Adnexa; Auditory System; Operating Microscope

Provide codes for the following procedures. Include any necessary modifiers. In some cases, more than one code is required.

1. removal of embedded foreign body, eyelid _____

2. biopsy, conjunctiva _____

3. ear piercing _____

4. removal, electromagnetic bone conduction hearing device, temporal bone

   _____

5. complete mastoidectomy _____

6. canthotomy _____

7. closure of eyelids by suture, temporary _____

8. scleral reinforcement without graft _____

9. extracapsular cataract removal with insertion of intraocular lens prothesis, mechanical technique

   _____

10. excision of scleral lesion _____

11. iridotomy by stab excision with transfixion _____

12. destruction of ciliary body by cryotherapy _____

13. repair of lacerated cornea with tissue glue _____

14. radial keratotomy _____

15. trabeculotomy ab externo _____

16. retinal detachment repaired with photocoagulation _____

17. recession procedure, strabismus surgery on one horizonal muscle

    _____

18. insertion of orbital implant _____

19. extraocular muscle chemodenervation _____

20. dacryocystotomy _____

21. removal of object from external auditory canal under general anesthesia

    _____

22. revision of stapedectomy _____

23. implanting a cochlear device _____

24. unlisted procedure of the middle ear _____

25. excision of eight lesions from the right eyelid _____

26. chalazion excision during the global period of a strabismus surgery

_____

27. tympanic membrane repair with operating microscope

_____

28. biopsy of both external ears _____

29. impacted cerumen removed from both ears _____

30. ocular implant removal with operating microscope _____

31. removal of dislocated intracapsular lens _____

32. discontinued myringoplasty _____

33. biopsy and excision of exostoses from external auditory canal

_____

34. tympanic neurectomy of both ears _____

35. canthus reconstruction, surgical care only _____

Radiology Section

Provide radiology codes for the following procedures. Do not include the -26 modifier. In some cases, more than one code is required.

1. radiologic examination of the ribs, two views (unilateral) _____

2. orthodontic cephalogram _____

3. magnetic resonance imaging of the pelvis with contrast _____

4. thoracic spine computerized tomography without contrast material

   _____

5. X ray examination of the abdomen, single anteroposterior view _____

6. antegrade urography, S&I _____

7. serialographic thoracic aortography, S&I _____

8. complete study, cardiac MRI for function _____

9. bilateral external carotid angiography, S&I _____

10. unilateral adrenal angiography, S&I _____

11. unilateral pelvic/abdominal lymphangiography, S&I _____

12. shoulder arthrography, S&I _____

13. fluoroscopic localization, needle biopsy _____

14. unilateral venography of extremity, S&I _____

15. pelvic CT with contrast material _____

16. ultrasonic foreign body localization, ophthalmic _____

17. transrectal echography _____

18. ultrasonic guidance, thoracentesis, S&I _____

19. simple therapeutic radiology treatment planning _____

20. intermediate brachytherapy isodose calculation _____

21. design and construction of complex customized shielding blocks, medical radiation treatment

   _____

22. radiation treatment management, eight treatments _____

23. hemibody irradiation _____

24. radiation treatment delivery, five areas, 20 MeV _____

25. 45 minutes physician time for fluoroscopy _____

26. CT bone density study and limited osseous survey _____

27. bilateral mammography _____

28. unlisted radiopharmaceutical therapeutic procedure _____

29. PET tumor imaging and metabolic evaluation _____

30. SPECT myocardial imaging _____

31. diagnostic nuclear medicine procedure, gastrointestinal, unlisted _____

32. ten determinations of thyroid uptake _____

33. high-intensity brachytherapy, remote afterloading, 11 catheters _____

34. repeated Doppler echocardiography, fetal cardiovascular system _____

35. transluminal atherectomy, S&I, three peripheral arteries _____

Pathology and Laboratory Section

Provide pathology and laboratory codes for the following procedures. Include any necessary modifiers. In some cases, more than one code is required.

Hint: Check the required components of the eleven organ/disease-oriented panels when coding multiple tests.

1. total serum cholesterol _____

2. blood creatinine _____

3. 3-specimen GTT _____

4. FSH gonadotropin test _____

5. 2 hours, gastric secretory study _____

6. Saccomanno technique _____

7. hepatitis C, direct probe _____

8. commercial-kit urine culture _____

9. Rh blood typing _____

10. EA test for Epstein-Barr virus _____

11. Chlamydia trachomatis infectious agent antigen detection, direct fluorescent antibody technique

    _____

12. stool test for Helicobacter pylori _____

13. reagent strip immunoassay for infectious agent antibody

    _____

14. bleeding time test _____

15. differential WBC count, buffy coat _____

16. complete CBC _____

17. ADH _____

18. Borrelia burgdoferi antibody _____

19. total testosterone _____

20. THBR uptake _____

21. total PSA _____

22. obstetric panel and lipid panel _____

23. lipid panel and triglycerides _____

24. ALT SGPT _____

25. Gram stain smear _____

26. urine specific gravity, automated, no microscopy _____

27. RPR, quantitative _____

28. potassium serum _____

29. hCG, quantitative _____

30. cholesterol, HDL, triglycerides, LDL _____

31. rubella screen _____

32. cryopreservation of five cell lines _____

33. HGH antibody _____

34. comprehensive clinical pathology consultation with report

    _____

35. mandated alcohol screen _____

Medicine Section

Provide medicine codes for the following procedures. Include any necessary modifiers. In many cases, more than one code is required.

1. subcutaneous injection of human rabies immune globulin

   _____

2. human immune globulin, intramuscular administration

   _____

3. intramuscular injection of Lyme disease vaccine _____

4. immunization with hepatitis A and hepatitis B vaccine

   _____

5. psychoanalysis _____

6. biofeedback training _____

7. hemodialysis procedure and single physician evaluation

   _____

8. diagnostic gastroenterology procedure, unlisted _____

9. fluorescein angiography _____

10. speech Stenger test _____

11. coronary thrombolysis by intracoronary infusion _____

12. PTCA _____

13. complete transthoracic echocardiography for congenital cardiac anomalies

    _____

14. limited transcranial Doppler study of intracranial arteries

    _____

15. total vital capacity _____

16. prick tests with allergenic extracts for (1) house dust, (2) seasonal grasses, (3) trees, (4) common

    ragweed, and (5) goldenrod _____

17. rapid desensitization procedure, discontinued _____

18. 2 hours, EEG monitoring _____

19. preparation of chemotherapy agent followed by arterial infusion, 3 hours

    _____

20. PUVA photochemotherapy _____

21. mandated occupational therapy re-evaluation _____

22. preparation and injections for allergies to bee and hornet stings

    _____

23. DTP and MMR vaccinations _____

24. IM injection of antibiotic _____

25. speech audiometry threshold test, one ear _____

26. percutaneous transluminal pulmonary artery balloon angioplasty, three arteries

    _____

Hint: Study the guidelines for cardiac catherization before coding these procedures.

27. right heart catheterization in the hospital _____

28. catheter placement for coronary angiography, in physician-owned catheterization laboratory

    _____

29. unusually complicated and difficult combined right heart and retrograde left heart catheterization

    _____

30. indicator dilution studies with arterial and venous catheterization, subsequent, in the hospital

    _____

31. percutaneous retrograde left heart catheterization from the femoral artery; injection procedure during the catheterization for aortography; and imaging supervision, interpretation, and report for

    aortography; in physician-owned cath laboratory _____

32. right heart catheterization and retrograde left heart catheterization for congenital anomalies, in the

    hospital _____

33. catheter placement in venous coronary bypass graft for coronary angiography; injection procedure for opacification of venous bypass graft; and imaging supervision, interpretation, and report; in

    physician-owned catheterization laboratory _____

HCPCS Level II National Codes and Modifiers

Provide HCPCS codes and modifiers for the following procedures.

1. standard wheelchair _____

2. adjustable semi-rigid cervical molded chin cup _____

3. Palmer WHFO _____

4. 12-volt Utah battery and battery charger _____

5. physical therapy evaluation and treatment, three visits _____

6. nonemergency BLS ambulance service _____

7. nasal cannula _____

8. occult blood test strips, for dialysis 100 _____

9. drainable ostomy pouch with attached barrier _____

10. levine type stomach tube _____

11. dysphagia screening _____

12. hearing aid fitting _____

13. anterior chamber intraocular lens _____

14. scratch resistant coating for a pair of glasses _____

15. cardiokymography _____

16. 2 mg, Dactinomycin _____

17. inhalation solution of Albuterol sulfate 0.5%, 2 ml, DME administration, unit dose

    _____

18. Isoetharine hydrochloride inhalation solution, DME administration, unit dose form, 1 milligram

    _____

19. routine venipuncture _____

20. multiple PET myocardial perfusion imaging following rest ECG _____

21. hemodialysis machine _____

22. electric hospital bed with mattress _____

23. pickup folding walker, new _____

24. nonsegmental home model, pneumatic compressor, rental _____

25. one gram of wound filler Hydrocolloid dressing, dry form _____

For the following, supply the CPT (HCPCS Level I) code or codes, as well as HCPCS modifiers, if appropriate.

26. excision of 1.0 benign lesion from upper right eyelid

    _____

27. release of thenar muscle, left thumb _____

28. acute chiropractic manipulative treatment, one spinal region

    _____

29. anesthesia for closed procedure in hip joint personally performed by anesthesiologist

    _____

30. ligation of anomalous left anterior descending coronary artery

    _____

31. hallux valgus correction, left foot, great toe _____

32. single determination, noninvasive pulse oximetry for oxygen saturation, technical component

    _____

33. extracapsular cataract extraction and insertion of IOL, performed in ambulatory surgical center

    _____

34. automated dip stick urinalysis, CLIA-waived test _____

35. closed treatment of acetabulum fracture with manipulation, right hip

    _____

Compliance

1. A patient of the Good Health Clinic asked the medical assistant to help her out of a tough financial spot. Her medical insurance authorized her to receive four radiation treatments for her condition, one every thirty-five days. Because she was out of town, she did not schedule her appointment for the last treatment until today, which is one week beyond the approved period. The insurance company will not reimburse the patient for this procedure. She asks the MA to change the date on the record to last Wednesday so that it will be covered, explaining that no one will be hurt by this change and, anyway, she pays the insurance company plenty.

   What type of action is the patient asking the MA to do?

   _____

   _____

   _____

   How should the MA handle the patient's request ?

   _____

   _____

   _____

2. What type of code edit could be used for the following rule? _____

   Medicare Part B covers a screening Pap smear for women for the early detection of cervical cancer but will not pay for an E/M service for the patient on the same day.

3. An OIG project found that during one month in a single state, there were 23,000 billings for an E/M service with the modifier -25 reported with one of these CPT-4 codes: 11055, 11056, 11057, 11719, and HCPCS code G0127 (trimming of dystrophic nails).

   Look up the descriptors for the CPT codes. Do you think the procedures appear to be simple or complicated?

   _____

   Why do you think that this billing combination continues to be under scrutiny by CMS?

   _____

Compliance Review

Match the key terms with the correct definitions.

A. upcode
B. NCCI edits
C. truncated coding
D. linkage
E. assumption coding

F. excluded parties
G. external audit
H. abuse
I. downcode
J. OIG Work Plan

_____ 1. A payer's review and reduction of a procedure code to a lower value than reported by the provider

_____ 2. The OIG's annual list of planned projects under the Medicare Fraud and Abuse Initiative

_____ 3. The connection between the service or procedure that was performed and the patient's condition or illness

_____ 4. Coding procedures that are not documented

_____ 5. An intentional act to deceive and take advantage of another person

_____ 6. A review of a practice's claims by an outside agent

_____ 7. Use of a procedure code that provides a higher reimbursement rate than the code for the service actually provided

_____ 8. A computerized screening system used to identify Medicare billing errors

_____ 9. Diagnosis codes that are not reported at the highest level of specificity available

_____10. The OIG's list of people/entities that are barred from Medicare work

Decide whether each statement is true or false, and write T for true or F for false.

_____11. Code linkage is analyzed to assess the patient's response to treatments.

_____12. The False Claims Act prohibits making a false statement to get a false claim paid by a government program.

_____13. Under Medicare rules, no modifiers can be used with code combinations listed in the CCI.

_____14. It is fraudulent to bill Medicare for a service that was not done.

_____15. Because the work was actually done, it is acceptable to change a date of service on a claim for a patient so that the charge is covered.

Write the letter of the choice that best completes the statement or answers the question.

_____ **16.** The OIG Work Plan describes
   A. planned projects for investigating possible fraud in various billing areas
   B. legislative initiatives under HIPAA
   C. the FBI's investigations
   D. the current cases that are being prosecuted by the OIG's attorneys

_____ **17.** Under Medicare's code edits, mutually exclusive codes
   A. can be billed together if they are component codes
   B. can be billed together if they have a -1 modifier code attached
   C. cannot be billed together for the same patient on the same day
   D. cannot be billed more than once by a single provider on the same date of service

_____ **18.** Intentionally reporting a service at a higher level than was performed is a clear example of
   A. auditing
   B. poor coding linkage
   C. assumption coding
   D. fraud

_____ **19.** Possible consequences of incorrect billing are
   A. downcoded claims
   B. upcoded claims
   C. unlinked claims
   D. code edits

_____ **20.** An encounter form containing E/M codes should list
   A. the most frequently billed codes
   B. just blanks, so the correct E/M code can be entered
   C. complete ranges of codes for each type or place of service listed
   D. none of the above

_____ **21.** If a coder selects codes on the basis of the documentation, the auditor's findings generally should _____ the coder's.
   A. disagree with
   B. agree with
   C. downcode
   D. have no relationship to

Analyze this case:

22. A forty-year-old established female patient is having an annual checkup. During the examination, her physician identifies a lump in her left breast. The physician considers this a significant finding and performs the key components of a problem-focused E/M service. These four codes and modifier should be reported. In what order should they be listed?

CPT codes: 99212, 99396

ICD codes: V70.0, 611.72

Modifier: -25

Verifying Linkage

The following diagnosis and procedure codes have been reported. In each case, indicate whether the codes are correctly linked ("Y" for yes) or not correctly linked ("N" for no).

	ICD-9-CM	CPT	LINKED?
1.	692.71	99201	_____
2.	410.01	99223	_____
3.	599.1	50600	_____
4.	216.1	67961	_____
5.	560.1	27147	_____
6.	766.2	99382	_____
7.	754.0	30520	_____
8.	250.51, 362.02	92012	_____
9.	733.81, 905.2	27824	_____
10.	568.0	56810	_____
11.	V76.12	76091	_____
12.	V54.8	99214	_____
13.	601.1, 041.1	57284	_____
14.	V58.1, 233.0	96408	_____
15.	824.2, 847.0, E888, E849.4	99203, 72040, 73600	_____

Selecting the Primary Diagnosis

Provide the diagnosis codes for the following statements. If sufficient information is given, also provide the procedure code. List the ICD-9-CM codes in the correct order, followed by the CPT codes.

1. severe abdominal pain, nausea, and vomiting from acute pancreatitis

   _____

2. vitamin B deficiency and sideroblastic anemia _____

3. cerebellar ataxia and hepatitis in chronic episodic alcoholism

   _____

4. pneumonia due to parainfluenza virus; radiologic examination of chest, special views

   _____

5. generalized peritonitis and acute appendicitis; appendectomy for ruptured appendix

   _____

6. direct ligation of esophageal varices due to portal hypertension

   _____

7. patient complained of hematuria and pyuria; urinalysis by bacterial culture of urine by commercial kit confirms acute pyelonephritis due to E. coli infection

   _____

8. physician performs cystourethroscopy with bilateral meatotomy to remove a foreign body in the

   genitourinary tract _____

9. postsurgical hypoglycemia and malnutrition; a breath hydrogen test is performed

   _____

10. due to dysmenorrhea and uterine endometriosis, physician performs a laparoscopic assisted vaginal

    hysterectomy, uterus less than 250 grams _____

Chronic or Undiagnosed Conditions

Provide the diagnosis codes for the following statements. If sufficient information is given, also provide the procedure code. List the ICD-9-CM codes in the correct order, followed by the CPT codes.

1. chronic and subacute arthropathy _____

2. encounter for chronic pleurisy with influenza _____

3. patient complains of blood in urine, frequent urination, and generalized abdominal pain; a tumor is suspected, and a diagnostic cystoscopy is scheduled

   _____

4. acute and chronic mesenteric lymphadenitis _____

5. vertigo; TIA suspected _____

6. pelvis swelling, probable malignant tumor _____

7. stereotactic needle core breast biopsy; finding of malignant primary tumor in upper-outer quadrant of left breast _____

8. routine 12-lead ECG with interpretation/report, abnormal finding

   _____

9. patient with chronic and acute maxillary sinusitis undergoes surgical nasal/sinus endoscopy and

   maxillary antrostomy _____

10. office consultation (comprehensive history and examination, moderately complex medical decision making) to evaluate complaints of nervousness, loss of sleep, and heat intolerance; diagnosis of

    thyrotoxicosis, rule out Graves' disease _____

V Codes and E Codes

Provide the diagnosis codes for the following statements. If sufficient information is given, also provide the procedure code. List the ICD-9-CM codes in the correct order, followed by the CPT codes.

1. single assay HIV-1 and HIV-2 screening test for AIDS; patient has no HIV-related symptoms

   _____

2. intramuscular injection of Hepatitis B globulin _____

3. annual medical examination of a 49-year-old male who is a new patient

   _____

4. bilateral screening mammography of patient whose mother and sister were diagnosed with breast

   cancer _____

5. normal vaginal delivery, antepartum/postpartum care, delivery of healthy boy

   _____

6. patient is a house painter who fell from scaffolding on the job and required closed treatment and

   manipulation of a humeral shaft fracture _____

7. local treatment of first-degree burns on both legs of an adult after clothing was burned by a bonfire

   _____

8. gastric intubation to remove stomach contents after patient was unconscious due to an accidental
   poisoning by an overdose of mescaline *Hint:* The diagnosis requires three codes—poisoning,

   manifestation, and cause. _____

9. office encounter with an established patient (expanded history/examination, low decision making
   complexity) who has nausea and vomiting due to an adverse reaction to an antibiotic

   _____

10. surgical exploration of a complicated chest wound caused by shotgun accident

    _____

Unspecified Diagnosis Codes

For each of the following diagnostic statements, what information is missing that would permit the assignment of a specific ICD-9-CM code?

1. patient complains of abdominal pain _____

2. gastric or intestinal hemorrhage _____

3. chronic bronchitis _____

4. acute myocardial infarction, location specified _____

5. chronic suppurative otitis media _____

6. acute reaction to stress _____

7. diabetes mellitus _____

8. monocytic leukemia in remission _____

9. streptococcus infection _____

10. osteoarthrosis _____

Surgical Diagnoses and Complications

Provide the diagnosis codes for the following statements. If sufficient information is given, also provide the procedure code. List the ICD-9-CM codes in the correct order, followed by the CPT codes. _Hint:_ Some procedures require the use of a modifier.

1. mechanical complication due to automatic implantable cardiac defibrillator

   _____

2. accidental puncture of the stomach during surgery

   _____

3. septicemia after repair of an open wound

   _____

4. vaccinia resulting from an immunization

   _____

5. complications arising after an incompatible blood transfusion

   _____

6. staphylococcus aureus septicemia due to an indwelling urinary catheter

   _____

7. during a procedure to implant a patient-activated cardiac event recorder, a hemorrhage occurs

   _____

8. 12 hours following surgery for an acute myocardial infarction, the electrode of a cardiac pacemaker fails, requiring additional surgery

   _____

9. following removal of a 2.5-cm tumor from the trunk of a patient, the pathology report indicates that it is malignant

   _____

10. a laparoscopic cholecystectomy is performed for a patient with acute cholecystitis; during the procedure, the patient has cardiac arrest, and after reviving of the patient, the surgeon terminates the procedure

    _____

Bundled (Global) Procedures and Laboratory Panels

Provide both the diagnostic and procedure codes for the following statements.

1. during an annual physical examination of a 62-year-old female established patient with a family history of kidney disease, the physician orders a comprehensive metabolic panel and a renal

   function panel _____

2. patient has blood in stool; physician performs a diagnostic sigmoidoscopy followed by removal of a

   foreign body _____

3. patient has a closed fracture of the tibial shaft; physician performs a closed treatment and applies

   an ambulatory short leg cast _____

4. following a biopsy, two benign sebaceous cystic skin lesions are excised—a 4.2 cm lesion from the hand of the patient and a 3.3 cm lesion from the patient's back; surgeon administered local

   anesthesia _____

5. patient has suffered an open fracture of multiple sites of her lower jaw bone when the car in which she was a passenger hit the highway divider; surgeon performs an open treatment that requires multiple approaches, including internal fixation, interdental fixation, and wiring of dentures

   _____

6. physician performs an endoscopically aided diagnostic bronchoscopy and a transbroncial lung biopsy under fluoroscopic guidance for a patient with pneumonia due to adenovirus

   _____

7. physician orders laboratory tests of total serum cholesterol, direct measurement of HDL cholesterol,

   and triglycerides for a patient with essential hypertension _____

8. elderly patient has been diagnosed with a mature cataract in the left eye; surgeon performs a one-stage extracapsular cataract removal with iridectomy, use of viscoelastic agents, and subconjunctival

   injections, and then inserts an intraocular lens prosthesis _____

9. patient has been diagnosed with carcinoma in situ of the prostate; surgeon performs a complete transurethral electrosurgical resection of the prostate; the procedure includes a vasectomy, meatotomy, cystourethroscopy, urethral calibration, and internal urethrotomy; control of

   postoperative bleeding is also required _____

10. after a comprehensive ophthalmological examination of a new Medicare patient, the ophthalmologist prescribes a corneal lens for the left eye; supplying the bifocal gas permeable

    contact lens is also reported _____

PART 5 Coding Quizzes

Coding Quiz: ICD-9-CM

Name/Class _____

_____ 1. Select the correct code for a personal history of cervical cancer:

    A. V16.41

    B. 180.9

    C. V10.41

    D. V10.40

_____ 2. Which is the correct code for a liveborn infant delivered by cesarean delivery in the hospital?

    A. V27.0

    B. V30.01

    C. V30

    D. V43.6

_____ 3. Select the correct code(s) for a patient who suffered an open fracture of the left radius in a fall from a moped on a highway.

    A. 813.05

    B. 813.91, E818.2

    C. 813.81, E818.0

    D. 813.91, E825.2

_____ 4. Light-headedness after taking a diazoxide prescription:

    A. 780.4, E942.5

    B. 386.9, E942.5

    C. 780.09

    D. 780.4

_____ 5. Select the correct code(s) for a plantar wart due to human papillomavirus infection.

    A. 078.19, 079

    B. 078.1

    C. 079.4

    D. 078.19, 079.4

_____ 6. Acute bulbar type I infantile paralysis:

    A. 045.0

    B. 045.9

    C. 045.01

    D. 045.91

_____ 7. Which code classifies preinvasive cancer of the female breast, upper-inner quadrant?

    A. 239.3

    B. 198.81

    C. 217

    D. 233.0

_____ 8. Screening test to rule out a suspected malignant neoplasm of the lung:

   A. V76.0
   B. V74.1
   C. V76.0, 162.9
   D. 162.9, V76.0

_____ 9. Select the correct code for chronic viral hepatitis B:

   A. 070.49
   B. 070.32
   C. 070.3
   D. 070

_____ 10. A patient has been diagnosed with Burkitt's tumor in the groin and the neck. Select the correct code(s).

   A. 200.8
   B. 200.25, 200.21
   C. 200.20
   D. 200.28

_____ 11. Select the correct code(s) for glaucoma and brittle type II diabetes.

   A. 250.00, 365.44
   B. 250.50
   C. 250.50, 365.44
   D. 250.40

_____ 12. Which of the following codes is correct for a diagnosis of abnormal coagulation profile?

   A. 790.92
   B. 286.9
   C. 286.90
   D. 776.0

_____ 13. Select the correct code for factor VIII deficiency.

   A. 286.4
   B. 286.0
   C. 286.2
   D. 286.3

_____ 14. Which of the following correctly codes senile dementia with confusion and depression?

   A. 290.0
   B. 290.2, 290.3
   C. 290.3, 290.21
   D. 290.41, 290.43

_____ 15. Select the correct code for recurrent manic-depressive disorder.

   A. 296.0
   B. 296.1
   C. 296.14
   D. 296. 10

_____ 16. Choose the code(s) that correctly describe meningitis due to St. Louis encephalitis.

    A. 321.2
    B. 321.2, 062.3
    C. 062.3, 321.2
    D. 323.4

_____ 17. Lesions of the lateral and medial popliteal nerves:

    A. 355.2
    B. 355.3, 355.4
    C. 724.3
    D. 353.3, 353.4

_____ 18. An elderly female patient has been diagnosed with glaucomatous subcapsular flecks and wide-angle glaucoma. Select the correct code(s).

    A. 365.10, 366.31
    B. 365.11
    C. 365.10
    D. 366.31, 365.10

_____ 19. A 43-year-old male patient receives a diagnosis of essential hypertension and chronic endocarditis. Choose the correct code(s).

    A. 401.1, 424.90
    B. 402.9, 424.90
    C. 410.0
    D. 401.9, 424.90

_____ 20. A 64-year-old female patient is readmitted to the hospital for evaluation of an acute myocardial infarction that occurred 3 weeks ago.

    A. 410.9
    B. 410.90
    C. 410.91
    D. 410.92

_____ 21. Select the correct code(s) for a diagnosis of acute influenzal myocarditis.

    A. 487.8, 422.0
    B. 422.0, 487.8
    C. 422.90, 487.8
    D. 487.8, 422.90

_____ 22. The patient's diagnosis is vesicoureteral reflux with nephropathy and chronic pyelonephritis due to Escherichia coli infection. Select the correct code(s).

    A. 593.70, 590.00, 041.4
    B. 590.00, 041.4
    C. 593.73, 590.00, 041.4
    D. 590.00, 041.4, 593.73

_____ 23. Purulent pleurisy with bronchocutaneous fistula due to a bacterial infection:

    A. 511.0, 041.9

    B. 510.0, 041.9

    C. 510.0

    D. 510.0, 510.9, 041.9

_____ 24. Choose the codes that properly classify ulcerative and acute gingivitis.

    A. 523.1, 523.0

    B. 523.4, 523.1

    C. 522.6, 523.0

    D. 523.0, 523.1

_____ 25. The patient is diagnosed with a recurrent gangrenous ventral hernia. Select the correct code(s).

    A. 551.21

    B. 553.21, 785.4

    C. 785.4, 553.21

    D. 551.21, 785.4

_____ 26. Diverticulosis and diverticulitis of the small intestine with bleeding:

    A. 562.01

    B. 562.03

    C. 562.01, 578.9

    D. 562.02, 562.03

_____ 27. A 58-year-old male patient has stenosis of the vesicourethral orifice and urinary incontinence. Select the correct code(s).

    A. 596.0, 625.6

    B. 596.0, 788.30

    C. 596.0

    D. 753.6, 788.30

_____ 28. A female infant 25 days old is light for her age, weighed 1200 grams at birth, and has dry peeling skin. Select the correct code(s).

    A. 764.14, 764.9

    B. 765.04

    C. 764.04

    D. 764.14

_____ 29. A pregnant patient in the twentieth week of gestation experiences bleeding:

    A. 640.9

    B. 640.90

    C. 640.95

    D. 640.80

_____ 30. Select the correct code(s) for acute pericardial effusion and chronic uremia.

    A. 420.0, 585

    B. 420.0, 586

    C. 585, 420.0

    D. 788.9

_____ 31. A patient's diagnosis is periostitis and acute osteomyelitis of the femur. Choose the correct code.

    A. 730.2

    B. 730.25

    C. 730.36

    D. 730.05

_____ 32. An infant is diagnosed with spina bifida and hydrocephalus; its spinal column at C1 and C2 did not close during fetal development. Which code is correct?

    A. 741.00

    B. 741.01

    C. 741.91

    D. 741.03

_____ 33. Eighteen hours following the delivery of her baby, a female patient suffers atonic hemorrhage. Choose the correct code.

    A. 666.1

    B. 666.0

    C. 666.14

    D. 666.10

_____ 34. A 24-year-old female patient has positive result from an HIV test; she is asymptomatic at the present. Which code is correct?

    A. 042

    B. V73.89

    C. V08

    D. V01.7

_____ 35. A patient presents to the emergency room in some distress, complaining of chest pain in the vicinity of the heart. The correct code is:

    A. 786.5

    B. 786.50

    C. 786.51

    D. 786.59

_____ 36. After an accident in which a car tire blows up, a patient suffers injuries to the saphenous vein and popliteal artery and vein. Select the correct codes.

    A. 904.3, 904.41, 904.42, E921.8

    B. 904.3, 904.40, E921.8

    C. E921.8, 904.3, 904.40

    D. 904.3, 904.41, 904.42

_____ 37. A patient experiences a superficial sunburn on the eyelids. Which codes are correct?

     A. 941.09, E926.2
     B. 941.12, E926.2
     C. 940.1, E926.2
     D. 692.71, E926.2

_____ 38. A patient has gastric hemorrhage following the ingestion of lye. Select the correct codes.

     A. 983.2, 578.9
     B. 983.2, 578.9, E980.6
     C. 578.9, 983.2
     D. 578.9, E980.6

_____ 39. After having acute poliomyelitis as a child, a patient experiences muscle weakness.

     A. 728.9, 138
     B. 138, 728.9
     C. 138
     D. 728.9

_____ 40. From a fire in a school, a patient has first-degree burns of the back of the hand and third-degree burns of the left foot. Which codes are correct?

     A. E891.8, 945.32, 944.16
     B. 945.32, 944.16, 948.21, E891.3
     C. 945.32, 944.16, 948.21
     D. 945.32, 944.16, E891.3

Coding Quiz: CPT

Name/Class _____

_____ 1. A cardiovascular surgeon begins to perform a percutaneous transcatheter placement of an intracoronary stent, but stops the procedure because of the patient's respiratory distress. Select the correct code.

    A. 92982
    B. 92980
    C. 92980-52
    D. 92980-53

_____ 2. A metal splinter was removed from the posterior segment of both eyes' ocular area using a magnet. Choose the correct code.

    A. 65260-52
    B. 65260-50
    C. 65235
    D. 65265

_____ 3. A surgeon performs a diagnostic ERCP and a trocar bladder aspiration. Which codes are correct?

    A. 43260, 51005-22
    B. 43260, 51005-51
    C. 43260, 51005-59
    D. 43260, 51005-62

_____ 4. A patient has an office encounter for removal of five skin tags on her hand. During the visit, she asks the physician to evaluate swelling and heat in her left knee. The physician performs an expanded history and examination with low medical decision making. What codes should be reported?

    A. 11200, 99214
    B. 11200, 99213-25
    C. 11100, 99213-25
    D. 11200, 99213-51

_____ 5. Following surgery to repair a sliding inguinal hernia, the patient is turned over to his primary care physician for all follow-up care. Which is the correct code for that follow-up care?

    A. 49525-55
    B. 49525-25
    C. 49525-77
    D. 49525-24

_____ 6. What is the correct code for a home visit with an established patient that required a detailed history of what has occurred since the physician's previous visit, a detailed examination, and moderately complex medical decision making?

    A. 99243
    B. 99343
    C. 99349
    D. 99313

_____ 7. A patient is referred to a specialist, who performs an E/M service in the office and prepares a written report for the referring physician. From what code range is the correct code chosen?

    A. 99241–99245

    B. 99251–99255

    C. 99261–99263

    D. 99271–99275

_____ 8. Selecting a code from the range for emergency department services depends on:

    A. whether the patient is new or established

    B. whether the patient is new or established, and what type of history is taken

    C. the type of history, examination, and medical decision making performed

    D. the type of history/examination performed and the amount of time spent

_____ 9. The physician is asked by the patient to perform a cardiovascular health risk assessment to evaluate his probability for heart disease. Which code is correct?

    A. 99401

    B. 99401-22

    C. 99272

    D. 99420

_____ 10. Modifier -47 is used for anesthesia services performed under difficult circumstances.

    A. True

    B. False

_____ 11. Which set of codes correctly describes the anesthesia services for insertion of a cardioverter/defibrillator via a transthoracic approach in a patient with severe systemic disease?

    A. 00534-P3

    B. 00560-P3

    C. 00534-P4

    D. 00560-P4

_____ 12. The correct code for a postoperative visit for the purpose of documentation is:

    A. 99070

    B. 99025

    C. 99024

    D. 99217

_____ 13. A global surgery code for a diagnostic procedure includes follow-up care related only to recovery from the procedure itself, not for care of the patient's underlying condition.

    A. True

    B. False

_____ 14. A patient's 3.9-cm benign lesion excision on the arm is followed by an intermediate repair involving a layered closure of 4.5 cm. Select the correct code(s).

    A. 11404

    B. 12002, 11424-51

    C. 12002, 11404-51

    D. 12032, 11404-51

_____ 15. A surgeon applied a 200-sq cm xenograft. The correct code(s) are:

A. 15400, 15401-51
B. 15400, 15401
C. 15350, 15351-58
D. 15050

_____ 16. A surgeon excised a chest wall tumor involving the ribs and then performed a mediastinal lymphadenectomy, followed by plastic reconstruction. Select the correct code(s).

A. 19160, 19162-51
B. 19260, 19272
C. 19272
D. 19260, 19272-51

_____ 17. After initiating a regional Bier block, a surgeon performs a closed treatment of an ulnar shaft fracture; the surgeon monitored the patient and the block during the surgery. Select the correct code(s) for this service.

A. 25530, 01820-47
B. 25530-47
C. 25530
D. 01820, 25530

_____ 18. Following the open treatment of a fractured big toe, the surgeon applies an ambulatory-type short leg cast. Choose the correct code(s).

A. 28515
B. 28525
C. 28505
D. 28505, 29425

_____ 19. A patient had a previous operation 15 days ago to treat a dislocated ankle. Today, the same surgeon repairs the patient's flexor tendon on the other foot. What code should be reported for today's service?

A. 28200-79
B. 28200
C. 28200-58
D. 28200-51

_____ 20. A physician removes a foreign body from a patient's nose during an office visit; local anesthesia was required. Should the anesthesia administration be reported for reimbursement?

A. Yes
B. No

_____ 21. Diagnostic endoscopy is performed on the left nasal cavity. Select the correct code.

A. 31237
B. 31231-52
C. 31231-50
D. 31231

_____ 22. Select the correct code(s) for a segmentectomy and bronchoplasty.

    A. 32484, 32501-51
    B. 32484, 32501
    C. 32484, 31770-51
    D. 32501

_____ 23. A cardiologist performs a second pericardiocentesis and provides supervision/interpretation of the radiological procedures. Choose the correct code(s).

    A. 33010
    B. 33010-26
    C. 33011, 76930
    D. 33011, 76930-26

_____ 24. Combined arterial and venous grafting for a coronary bypass is coded using the range 33517–33523.

    A. True
    B. False

_____ 25. The repair of a ruptured aneurysm of the abdominal aorta is made extremely complicated by the patient's obesity; the procedure takes twice as long as normally anticipated, which is appropriately documented in the operative report. Select the correct code.

    A. 35001
    B. 35082-21
    C. 35082
    D. 35082-22

_____ 26. Following a diagnostic thoracoscopy and biopsy of the mediastinal space, the surgeon performs a surgical thorascopy and excises a mediastinal mass. Select the correct code(s).

    A. 32606, 32662-51
    B. 32606, 32662-59
    C. 32662
    D. 32601, 32606

_____ 27. The correct reporting of a separate procedure that is not done as part of a surgical package requires which of the following modifiers?

    A. -51
    B. -54
    C. -59
    D. -99

_____ 28. The correct code for a laparoscopically aided esophagogastric fundoplasty is 43280. What is the code for the same procedure using an open approach?

    A. 43289
    B. 43324
    C. 43325
    D. 49320

_____ 29. A surgeon performs a modified radical mastectomy, including the axillary lymph nodes, following an incisional breast biopsy which resulted in a finding of malignancy. Select the correct code(s) for these procedures.

    A. 19240, 19101
    B. 19240, 19101-51
    C. 19240
    D. 19240-52

_____ 30. A cesarean delivery followed an attempted vaginal delivery. The mother's previous children had been born with cesarean delivery. The physician handled both the delivery and routine antepartum and postpartum care. Select the correct code.

    A. 59618
    B. 59620
    C. 59622
    D. 59610

_____ 31. The surgeon created a twist drill hole for subdural puncture in order to implant a pressure recording device. Select the correct code(s).

    A. 61105, 61107-51
    B. 61105, 61107-59
    C. 61105, 61107
    D. 61107

_____ 32. Many radiology procedures have two parts:
    A. unlisted or guided
    B. supervision or interpretation
    C. professional or technical
    D. complete or partial

_____ 33. The correct code for the supervision and interpretation of a selective, unilateral angiography of an external carotid artery is:

    A. 75660-26
    B. 75662-26
    C. 75660
    D. 75662

_____ 34. Select the correct code(s) for these laboratory tests: carbon dioxide, sodium, urea nitrogen, creatinine, chloride, calcium, glucose, and potassium.

    A. 82374, 84295, 84520, 82565, 82435, 82310, 82947, 84132
    B. 80051, 82310, 82565, 84520
    C. 80053
    D. 80048

_____ 35. A growth hormone stimulation panel and an aldosterone test are ordered. Choose the correct codes.

    A. 80428, 82088-51
    B. 80428, 82088
    C. 80428, 82088-59
    D. 80435, 82088

_____ 36. An intravenous injection of immune globulin, 1 g, is administered to a Medicare patient. Which code(s) are correct?

    A. 90283, 90784
    B. 90281, 90782
    C. J1563, 90784
    D. J1561

_____ 37. A cardiologist performs a percutaneous retrograde left heart cardiac catheterization from the femoral artery requiring left atrial angiography. The cardiologist provided imaging supervision, interpretation, and report. Select the correct codes.

    A. 93511, 93542, 93561
    B. 93542, 93555
    C. 93510, 93543, 93555-26
    D. 93510, 93543, 93556

_____ 38. To study a patient's sleep disorder, a neurologist conducted an extended 4-hour monitoring of the patient's EEG. Choose the correct code.

    A. 95812
    B. 95813
    C. 95813-22
    D. 95816

_____ 39. For a Medicare patient, which range of codes is used for prosthetic procedures?

    A. L5000–L8699
    B. M0064–M0302
    C. J0120–J8999
    D. A4206–A6406

_____ 40. A Medicare patient is prescribed a wheelchair with detachable arms and leg rests. Which code is correct?

    A. E1050
    B. E1083
    C. E1150
    D. E1160

Coding Quiz: Coding Linkage and Compliance

Name/Class _____

_____ 1. Which of the following is **not** required for correctly linked codes?

    A. The diagnosis and procedure codes present a logical clinical relationship.

    B. The diagnosis and procedures codes are from the same data set.

    C. The procedures are necessary and effective, and are not elective or experimental.

    D. The treatment is provided at an appropriate level for the presenting problem.

_____ 2. In the diagnostic statement "eye dryness and irritation from insufficient tear production," the primary diagnosis is:

    A. eye dryness

    B. eye irritation

    C. tear production

    D. insufficient tear production

_____ 3. The patient presents with transient infiltrations of the lungs by eosinophilia, resulting in cough, fever, and dyspnea. Select the correct diagnosis code(s).

    A. 786.2, 780.6

    B. 780.6, 786.2

    C. 518.3

    D. 786.9

_____ 4. Computerd axial tomography without contrast is performed on the maxillofacial area for a patient with chronic sinusitis. Select the correct diagnosis and procedure codes.

    A. 473, 70486

    B. 473.0, 70486

    C. 473.9, 70486

    D. 473.8, 70486

_____ 5. An inconclusive diagnosis is indicated by terms such as:

    A. rule out, suspected, probable

    B. finding, result, report

    C. malignant, benign, in situ

    D. adverse effect, poisoning, unspecified

_____ 6. Following catheterization and introduction of contrast material, a hysterosonographic study with radiological supervision and interpretation is conducted for a patient with postmenopausal bleeding and suspected endometrial carcinoma. Select the correct diagnosis and procedure codes.

    A. 239.5, 58350, 76831

    B. 182.0, 58340, 76831-26

    C. 627.1, 58340, 76831-26

    D. 627.1, 182.0, 58340, 76831

7. A biopsy of a dark growth on the back of a patient's hand reported a finding of a 0.9-cm malignant lesion, which was excised under local anesthesia. Select the correct diagnosis and procedure codes.

   A. 195.4, 17261-47
   B. 195.4, 17261
   C. 709.9, 11621
   D. 195.4, 11621

8. Select the correct codes for an annual physical examination of a 4-year-old established patient.

   A. V70.0, 99392
   B. V20.2, 99392
   C. V70.0, 99382
   D. V70.3, 99401

9. Following exposure to possible rabies from a dog bite, the patient is inoculated intramuscularly with a rabies vaccine. Choose the correct codes.

   A. V04.5, E906.0, 90675, 90471
   B. E906.0, V01.5, 90675, 90471
   C. V01.5, E906.0, 90675, 90471
   D. V01.5, E906.0, 90675, 90782

10. Both V codes and E codes may be primary or secondary, depending on the circumstances involved.

   A. True
   B. False

11. Select the correct diagnosis code for the following statement: "The patient suffers from atherosclerotic heart disease caused by plaque deposits in a grafted internal mammary artery. The patient underwent this arterial bypass graft procedure 4 months ago."

   A. 414.0
   B. 414.01
   C. 414.04
   D. 414.9

12. When the physician owns the equipment and provides the supplies and technical service when providing radiology procedures, the -26 modifier is not appropriate.

   A. True
   B. False

13. After introduction of anesthesia for an intracranial vascular procedure, the patient suddenly went into respiratory distress and the procedure was terminated. What is the correct code?

   A. 00216-53
   B. 00216
   C. 00210-53
   D. 61105-53

_____ 14. In most cases, a biopsy of a site performed with a definitive procedure such as an excision or surgical removal of an organ is not coded.

   A. True
   B. False

_____ 15. A patient had a total abdominal hysterectomy 35 days ago and has had increasing pain in the area of the incision. The surgeon performs a diagnostic laparoscopy and, finding adhesions, performs a surgical lysis. Select the correct codes.

   A. 182.1, 58200
   B. 614.6, 58660
   C. 182.1, 58660-78
   D. 614.6, 58660-78

_____ 16. As part of a routine physical examination of a 70-year-old female Medicare patient who sees the doctor every year, the primary care physician orders tests of total serum cholesterol, HDL cholesterol, and triglycerides, and also administers an cytomegalovirus human immune globulin injection. Select the correct codes for the physician's work and the laboratory services.

   A. V70.0, 99397, G0001, 82465, 83718, 84478, 90291, 90784
   B. V70.0, 99397, G0001, 80061, 90291, 90784
   C. V70.0, 99397, G0001, 80061, J0850, 90784
   D. V70.0, 99397, G0001, 80061, 90291, 90781

_____ 17. A patient has a chronic ulcer of the lower limb. During an initial operation, the surgeon prepares the site of the ulcer and uses an allograft to permit healing. Thirty days later, the patient is returned to the OR for a free skin flap. What are the correct codes for the second operation?

   A. 707.1, 15757
   B. 707.10, 15757-58
   C. 707.8, 15757-59
   D. 707.1, 15757-76

_____ 18. A surgeon performs a peritoneoscopy to diagnose reported pain in the right lower quadrant of the patient's abdomen. Based on the findings, the surgeon schedules the patient for a surgical laparoscopic procedure to remove a follicular ovarian cyst. Is the diagnostic procedure included in the surgical procedure in this case?

   A. Yes
   B. No

_____ 19. After seeing the patient in the office, the physician admits her for observation. In the hospital, the physician performs a comprehensive history and examination, decision making of high complexity, and decides to schedule the patient for surgery. What procedure code is appropriate?

   A. 99220
   B. 99223-57
   C. 99291
   D. 99220-57

_____ 20. An obstetrician providing routine antepartum, delivery, and postpartum care performs amniocentesis during the first trimester of the patient's pregnancy. Based on CPT-4, is this service included in the global obstetric package?

   A. Yes
   B. No

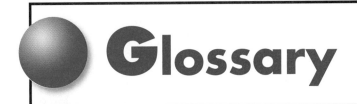 Glossary

A

abuse Actions that improperly use another's resources.

Acknowledgment of Receipt of Notice of Privacy Practices Form accompanying a covered entity's Notice of Privacy Practices; covered entities must make a good-faith effort to have patients sign the acknowledgment.

acute Describes an illness or condition having severe symptoms and a short duration; can also refer to a sudden exacerbation of a chronic condition.

addenda Updates to the ICD-9-CM diagnostic coding system.

add-on code Procedures that are performed and reported only in addition to a primary procedure; indicated in CPT by a plus sign (+) next to the code.

admitting diagnosis The patient's condition determined by a physician at admission to an inpatient facility.

adverse effect Condition due to the correct usage of a drug.

Alphabetic Index The section of the ICD-9-CM in which diseases and injuries with corresponding diagnosis codes are presented in alphabetical order.

ambulatory care Outpatient care.

American Academy of Professional Coders (AAPC) National association that fosters the establishment and maintenance of professional, ethical, education, and certification standards for medical coding.

American Association of Medical Assistants National association that fosters the profession of medical assisting.

American Association for Medical Transcription National association fostering the profession of medical transcription.

American Health Information Management Association (AHIMA) National association of health information management professionals; promotes valid, accessible, yet confidential health information and advocates quality health care.

American Medical Association (AMA) Member organization for physicians; goals are to promote the art and science of medicine, improve public health, and promote ethical, educational, and clinical standards for the medical profession.

assumption coding Reporting undocumented services that the coder assumes have been provided because of the nature of the case or condition.

attending physician The clinician primarily responsible for the care of the patient from the beginning of a hospitalization.

audit Methodical review; in medical insurance, a formal examination of a physician's accounting or patient medical records.

B

bundled code Single procedure code used to report a group of related procedures.

C

CMS See Centers for Medicare and Medicaid Services.

CMS-1450 Paper claim for hospital services; also known as the UB-92.

CMS-1500 Paper claim for physician services.

CPT   The abbreviation that refers to the American Medical Association's publication *Current Procedural Terminology.*

carrier   Health plan; also known as insurance company, payer, or third-party payer.

category   In the ICD-9-CM, a three-digit code used to classify a particular disease or injury.

Category I codes   The codes for evaluation and management, surgical, pathology/laboratory, radiology, and medical services in CPT.

Category II codes   Optional CPT codes that track performance measures for a medical goal such as reducing tobacco use.

Category III codes   Temporary codes for emerging technology, services, and procedures; to be used, rather than a unlisted code, when available.

Centers for Medicare and Medicaid Services (CMS)   Federal agency within the Department of Health and Human Services (HHS) that runs Medicare, Medicaid, Clinical Laboratories (under the CLIA program), and other governmental health programs.

chief complaint (CC)   A patient's description of the symptoms or other reasons for seeking medical care for a provider encounter.

chronic   An illness or condition with a long duration.

code edits   A computerized screening system used to identify improperly or incorrectly reported codes.

code linkage   The connection between a service and a patient's condition or illness; establishes the medical necessity of the procedure.

code set   Alphabetic and/or numeric representations for data. Medical code sets are systems of medical terms that are required for HIPAA transactions. Administrative (non-medical) code sets, such as taxonomy codes and Zip codes, are also used in HIPAA transactions.

coding   The process of assigning numerical codes to diagnoses and procedures/services.

coexisting condition   Additional illness that either has an effect on the patient's primary illness or is also treated during the encounter.

combination code   A single code that classifies both the etiology and the manifestation of an illness or injury.

comorbidity   Admitted patient's coexisting condition which affects the length of the hospital stay or the course of treatment.

compliance plan   A medical practice's written plan for (a) the appointment of a compliance officer and committee, (b) a code of conduct for physicians' business arrangements and employees' compliance, (c) training plans, (d) properly prepared and updated coding tools such as job reference aids, encounter forms, and documentation templates, (e) rules for prompt identification and refunding of overpayments, and (f) ongoing monitoring and auditing of claim preparation.

complication   Condition an admitted patient develops after surgery or treatment that affects the length of hospital stay or the course of further treatment.

concurrent care   Medical situation in which a patient receives extensive, independent care from two or more attending physicians on the same date of service.

consultation   Service performed by a physician to advise a requesting physician about a patient's condition and care; the consultant does not assume responsibility for the patient's care and must send a written report back to the requestor.

convention   Typographic techniques or standard practices that provide visual guidelines for understanding printed material.

Correct Coding Initiative See **National Correct Coding Initiative.**

counseling   Physician's discussion with a patient and/or family concerning diagnostic results, prognosis, treatment options, and/or instructions.

cross-reference   Directions in printed material that tell a reader where to look for additional information.

crosswalk   A comparison or map of the codes for the same or similar classifications under two coding systems that provides a guide for selecting the closest match.

Current Procedural Terminology (CPT) Publication of the American Medical Association containing the HIPAA-mandated standardized classification system for reporting medical procedures and services performed by physicians.

D

descriptor   The narrative part of a CPT code that identifies the procedure or service.

diagnosis   A physician's opinion of the nature of a patient's illness or injury.

diagnosis code   The number assigned to a diagnosis in the *International Classification of Diseases.*

diagnostic statement   A physician's description of the main reason for a patient's encounter; may also describe related conditions or symptoms.

documentation   The systematic, logical, and consistent recording of a patient's health status—history, examinations, tests, results of treatments, and observations—in chronological order in a patient medical record.

documentation template   Physician practice form used to prompt the physician to document a complete review of systems (ROS) when done and the medical necessity for the planned treatment.

downcode   A payer's review and reduction of a procedure code (often an E/M code) to a lower level than reported by the provider.

durable medical equipment (DME)   Medicare term for reusable physical supplies such as wheelchairs and hospital beds that are ordered by the provider for use in the home; reported with HPCPS Level II codes.

E

E code   An alphanumeric ICD code for an external cause of injury or poisoning.

E/M   See evaluation and management code.

elective surgery   Non-emergency surgical procedure that can be scheduled in advance.

emergency   A situation in which a delay in the treatment of the patient would lead to a significant increase in the threat to life or body part.

encounter   An office visit between a patient and a medical professional.

encounter form   A listing of the diagnoses, procedures, and charges for a patient's visit; also called the superbill.

eponym   A name or phrase that is formed from or based on a person's name; usually describes a condition or procedure associated with that person.

established patient   A patient who has received professional services from a provider (or another provider with the same specialty in the same practice) within the past three years.

etiology   The cause or origin of a disease.

evaluation and management (E/M) codes Procedure codes that cover physicians' services performed to determine the optimum course for patient care; listed in the Evaluation and Management section of CPT.

excluded parties   Individuals/companies who, because of reasons bearing on professional competence, professional performance, or financial integrity, are not permitted by the OIG to participate in any federal health care programs.

external audit   Audit conducted by an organization outside of the practice, such as a federal agency.

F

formulary   A list of a health plan's selected drugs and their proper dosages.

fragmented billing   Incorrect billing practice in which procedures covered under a single bundled code are "unbundled" and separately reported.

fraud   Intentional deceptive act to obtain a benefit.

G

gatekeeper   See primary care physician.

global period   The number of days surrounding a surgical procedure during which all services relating to the procedure—preoperative, during the surgery, and postoperative—are considered part of the surgical package and are not additionally reimbursed.

global surgical concept   See surgical package.

H

HCFA   See Centers for Medicare and Medicaid Services.

Health Care Financing Administration   See Centers for Medicare and Medicaid Services.

Healthcare Common Procedure Coding System (HCPCS)   Procedure codes for Medicare claims, made up of CPT codes (Level I) and national codes (Level II).

Health Care Fraud and Abuse Control Program   Government program to uncover misuse of funds in federal health care programs; run by the Office of the Inspector General (OIG).

Health Insurance Portability and Accountability Act (HIPAA) of 1996   Federal act that set forth guidelines for standardizing the electronic data interchange of administrative and financial transactions, exposing fraud and abuse in government programs, and protecting the security and privacy of health information.

health plan   Under HIPAA, an individual or group plan that either provides or pays for the cost of, medical care, including group health plan, health insurance issuer, health maintenance organization, Medicare Part A or B, Medicaid, TRICARE, and other governmental and nongovernmental plans.

HIPAA claim   Generic term for the HIPAA ASC X12N 837 professional health care claim transaction.

I

ICD-9-CM   Abbreviated title of International Classification of Diseases, 9th Revision, Clinical Modification.

ICD code   A system of diagnostic codes based on the International Classification of Diseases.

incident-to   Term for services of allied health professionals, such as nurses, technicians, and therapists, provided under the physician's supervision that may be billed under Medicare.

inpatient   A person admitted to a medical facility for services that require an overnight stay.

internal audit   A self-audit conducted by a staff member or consultant as a routine check of compliance with reporting regulations.

International Classification of Diseases, 9th Revision, Clinical Modification (ICD-9-CM)   A publication containing the HIPAA-mandated standardized classification system for diseases and injuries; developed by the World Health Organization and modified for use in the United States.

J

job reference aid   A list of a medical practice's frequently reported procedures and diagnoses.

L

late effect   Condition that remains after an acute illness or injury has completed its course.

M

M code   A classification number that identifies the morphology of neoplasms.

main number The five-digit procedure code listed in the CPT.

main term The word in bold-faced type that identifies a disease or condition in the Alphabetic index in ICD-9-CM.

manifestation A characteristic sign or symptom of a disease.

medical error Failure of a planned action to be completed as intended or the use of a wrong plan to achieve an aim. Errors that result in patient harm are "adverse effects," those that did not are "near misses." The most common form of errors is drug errors.

medical malpractice Failure to use an acceptable level of professional skill when giving medical services that results in injury or harm to a patient.

medical necessity Payment criterion of payers that requires medical treatments to be appropriate and provided in accordance with generally accepted standards of medical practice. The reported procedure or service (1) matches the diagnosis, (2) is not elective, (3) is not experimental, (4) has not been performed for the convenience of the patient or the patient's family, and (5) has been provided at the appropriate level.

medical record A file that contains the documentation of a patient's medical history, record of care, progress notes, correspondence, and related billing/financial information.

medical terminology The terms used to describe diagnoses and procedures; based on anatomy.

Medicare carrier A private organization under contract with CMS to administer Medicare claims in an assigned region.

modifier A number that is appended to a code to report particular facts. CPT modifiers report special circumstances involved with a procedure or service. HCPCS modifiers are often used to designate a body part, such as left side or right side.

moribund Approaching death.

multiple modifiers Two or more modifiers used to augment a procedure code.

N

National Correct Coding Initiative (NCCI) Computerized Medicare system to prevent overpayment for procedures.

National Correct Coding Initiative edits Pairs of CPT or HCPCS Level II codes that are not separately payable by Medicare except under certain circumstances. The edits apply to services by the same provider for the same beneficiary on the same date of service.

new patient A patient who has not received professional services from a provider (or another provider with the same specialty in the same practice) within the past three years.

not elsewhere classified (NEC) An ICD-9-CM abbreviation indicating the code to be used when an illness or condition cannot be placed in any other category.

not otherwise specified (NOS) An ICD-9-CM abbreviation indicating the code to be used when no information is available for assigning the illness or condition a more specific code.

O

Office of the Inspector General (OIG) Government agency that investigates and prosecutes fraud against government health care programs such as Medicare.

OIG Compliance Program Guidance for Individual and Small Group Physician Practices OIG publication that explains the recommended features of compliance plans for small providers.

OIG Work Plan The OIG's annual list of planned projects under the Medicare Fraud and Abuse Initiative.

outpatient A patient who receives health care in a hospital setting without admission; the length of stay is generally less than 23 hours.

P

panel   In CPT, a single code grouping laboratory tests that are frequently done together.

patient information form   A form that includes a patient's personal, employment, and insurance company data needed to complete a health care claim; also known as a registration form.

physical status modifier   A code used in the Anesthesia Section of CPT with procedure codes to indicate the patient's health status.

preexisting condition   An illness or disorder of a beneficiary that existed before the effective date of insurance coverage.

preventive medical services   Care that is provided to keep patients healthy or to prevent illness, such as routine checkups and screening tests.

primary care physician (PCP)   A physician who directs all aspects of a patient's care, including routine services, referrals to specialists within the system, and supervision of hospital admissions; also known as a gatekeeper.

primary diagnosis   A diagnosis that represents the patient's major illness or condition for an encounter.

primary procedure   The most resource-intensive (highest paid) CPT procedure done during a patient's encounter.

principal diagnosis   The condition that after study is established as chiefly responsible for a patient's admission to a hospital.

principal procedure   The main service performed for the condition listed as the principal diagnosis for a hospital inpatient.

procedure code   A code that identifies medical treatment or diagnostic services.

professional component   The part of the relative value associated with a procedure code that represents a physician's skill, time, and expertise used in performing it; as opposed to the technical component.

prognosis   The physician's prediction of outcome of disease and likelihood of recovery.

provider   A person or entity that supplies medical or health services and bills for or is paid for the services in the normal course of business. A provider may be a professional member of the health care team, such as a physician, or a facility, such as a hospital or skilled nursing home.

R

referral   Transfer of patient care from one physician to another.

referral number   Authorization number given by a referring physician to the referred physician.

referring provider   The physician who refers the patient to another physician for treatment.

respondeat superior   Doctrine making the employer responsible for employees' actions.

S

SOAP *Subjective/Objective/Assessment/Plan* Documentation format in which encounter information is grouped into four sections containing the patient's subjective descriptions of signs and symptoms; the physician's notes on the objective information regarding the condition and examination/test results; the physician's assessment, or diagnosis, of the condition; and the plan of treatment.

secondary condition   Additional diagnosis(ses) that occurs at the same time as a primary diagnosis and that affects its treatment.

secondary procedure   A procedure performed in addition to the primary procedure.

section guidelines   Usage notes provided at the beginnings of CPT sections.

separate procedure   Descriptor used in the Surgery Section of CPT for a procedure that is usually part of a surgical package but may also be performed separately or for a different purpose, in which case it may be reported separately.

special report   A note prepared to detail the reasons for a new, variable, or unlisted procedure or service; explains the patient' condition and justifies the procedure's medical necessity.

subcategory   In ICD-9-CM, a four-digit code number.

subclassification   In ICD-9-CM, a five-digit code number.

subterm   A word or phrase that describes a main term in the Alphabetic Index of the ICD-9-CM.

superbill   A listing of the diagnoses, procedures, and charges for a patient's visit; also called the encounter form.

supplementary term   A nonessential word or phrase that helps to define a code in the ICD-9-CM; usually enclosed in parentheses or brackets.

surgical package   A combination of services included in a single procedure code for some surgical procedures in CPT.

T

Tabular List   The section of the ICD-9-CM in which diagnosis codes are presented in numerical order.

technical component   The part of the relative value associated with a procedure code that reflects the technician's work and the equipment and supplies used in performing it; as opposed to professional component.

truncated coding   Diagnoses that are not coded at the highest level of specificity available.

U

UB-92   Paper hospital claim; also known as the CMS-1450.

unbundling   The incorrect billing practice of breaking a panel or package of services/ procedures into component parts and reporting them separately.

unlisted procedure   A service that is not listed in CPT; reported with an unlisted procedure code and requires a special report when used.

unspecified   An incompletely described condition which must be coded with an unspecified ICD code.

upcode   Use of a procedure code that provides a higher payment than the code for the service actually provided.

V

V code   An alphanumeric code in the ICD-9-CM that identifies factors that influence health status and encounters that are not due to illness or injury.

Index

Hemic system, CPT Surgery coding for, 67

High blood pressure, ICD-9-CM coding for, 26–27, 29

History of present illness (HPI), 52

HIV/AIDS, ICD-9-CM coding for, 29

Hospital care, outpatient or ambulatory, 17, 18–19, 55, 56–57

HPI (history of present illness), 52

Hypertension, ICD-9-CM coding for, 26–27, 29

Hypertensive heart disease, ICD-9-CM coding for, 26–27

I

ICD-9-CM codes, 4–33
  addenda, 4, 5
  Alphabetic Index, 5, 6–9
    abbreviations, 8
    common terms, 9
    cross-references, 7–8
    eponyms, 9
    locating primary diagnosis in, 17
    main terms, 6
    M (morphology) codes, 24
    multiple codes and connecting words, 8–9
    Neoplasm Table, 23–24
    notes, 8
    subterms, 6
    supplementary terms, 6–7, 9, 14–16
    turnover lines, 7
  annual updates, 4, 5, 90
  cheat sheets, 91
  coding guidelines, 17–23
    coexisting conditions, 20
    highest level of certainty, 21–22
    highest level of specificity, 22–23
    primary diagnosis, 17, 20, 92–93
    surgery codes, 22
  coding steps, 6, 16–17
  linkage between CPT codes and, 84, 87–88, 92
  nature of, 4
  new revision, ICD-10-CM, 5
  organization of, 5–6
  origins of, 4
  specific diagnoses, 22–32
    acute versus chronic conditions, 21
    blood and blood-forming organ diseases, 25
    burns, 30–31
    circulatory diseases, 26–27, 29
    coding to highest level of specificity, 22–23
    congenital anomalies, 28
    connective tissue diseases, 28
    digestive system diseases, 27
    endocrine diseases, 25
    fractures, 29–30

    genitourinary system diseases, 27
    high blood pressure, 26–27, 29
    HIV/AIDs, 29
    ill-defined conditions, 29
    immunity disorders, 25
    infectious and parasitic diseases, 23
    injury and poisoning, 29–32
    late effects, 21, 32
    mental disorders, 25–26
    metabolic diseases, 25
    musculoskeletal system diseases, 28
    neoplasms, 23–24
    nervous system and sense organ diseases, 26
    nutritional diseases, 25
    perinatal period conditions, 29
    poisoning versus adverse effects, 32
    pregnancy, childbirth, and puerperium complications, 28
    respiratory system diseases, 27
    skin and subcutaneous tissue diseases, 28
  Tabular List, 5, 6, 9–14
    abbreviations, 13
    categories, 9, 10
    fifth-digit requirement, 11–12, 23
    multiple codes, 13–14
    notes, 12
    punctuation, 12–13, 25
    sample entries, 11
    subcategory, 10
    subclassification, 11
    supplementary classifications, 14–16
    symbols, 11–12
    verifying code in, 17

ICD-10-CM codes, 5

Ill-defined conditions, ICD-9-CM coding for, 29

Immunity disorders, ICD-9-CM coding for, 25

Immunizations, CPT (E/M) codes, 73

Incident-to billing, 84

Indentions (CPT), 42

Infectious diseases, ICD-9-CM coding for, 23

Integumentary system, CPT Surgery coding for, 66

Internal audits, 90

International Classification of Diseases, Ninth Revision, *Clinical Modification* (ICD-9-CM), 4–33

Ischemic heart disease, ICD-9-CM coding for, 26

J

Job reference aids (cheat sheets), 91

L

Late effects, ICD-9-CM coding for, 21, 32

Linkage and compliance review, 84, 87–88, 92

List of Excluded Individuals/Entities (LEIE), 85

Lozenge (ICD-9-CM), 13

Lymphatic system, CPT Surgery coding for, 67

M

Main terms
    CPT, 38
    ICD-9-CM, 6
Male genital system, CPT Surgery coding for, 67
Manifestation, 9, 93
Maternity care
    CPT Surgery coding for, 68
    ICD-9-CM coding for complications, 28
M (morphology) codes, 24
Mediastinum, CPT Surgery coding for, 67
Medical liability insurance, 89
Medical necessity review, coding errors relating
    to, 87–88
Medicare
    claim preparation and processing
        HCPCS codes required for, 36, 73, 74–77
        ICD-9 codes required for, 4
        National Correct Coding Initiative
            (NCCI), 85–86
        regulations and requirements, 85–86
    fraud detection and investigation, 82–83,
        85–86
Medicare carriers, 84, 86
Medicare Catastrophic Coverage Act (1988), 4
Medicine codes (CPT), 37, 72–73, 79
    reporting, 73
    structure and modifiers, 72–73
Mental disorders, ICD-9-CM coding for, 25–26
Metabolic diseases, ICD-9-CM coding for, 25
Modifiers
    CPT, 38, 44–47
        Anesthesia codes, 58–60
        bilateral, 64
        determining need for, 46–47
        Evaluation and Management (E/M) codes,
          51, 56
        listing of, 44–45
        Medicine codes, 72–73
        Pathology and Laboratory codes, 71, 94
        procedures exempt from -51 modifier, 69
        Radiology codes, 70–71
        reporting, 46–47
        Surgical section, 63–65
        use of, 46–47
    HCPCS codes, 76–77
Multiple codes (ICD-9-CM), 8–9
    code also, 14
    code first underlying disease, 13
    use additional code, 14
    use additional code, if desired, 14
Musculoskeletal system
    CPT Surgery coding for, 66
    ICD-9-CM coding for diseases of, 28
    ICD-9-CM coding for fractures, 29–30

N

National Center for Health Statistics (NCHS),
    4–5, 17
National Correct Coding Initiative (NCCI),
    85–86
NCCI edits, 85–86
NEC (not elsewhere classified), 8, 13, 25
Neoplasms, ICD-9-CM coding for, 23–24
Nervous system
    CPT Surgery coding for, 68
    ICD-9-CM coding for diseases of, 26
New patients, Evaluation and Management
    (E/M) codes, 49–50
NOS (not otherwise specified), 13, 25
Not elsewhere classified (NEC), 8, 13, 25
Notes (ICD-9-CM), 8, 12
Not otherwise specified (NOS), 13, 25
Nutritional diseases, ICD-9-CM coding for, 25

O

Occupational Safety and Health Administration
    (OSHA), 72
Office of the Inspector General (OIG), 84–85
OIG Work Plan, 84
OSHA (Occupational Safety and Health
    Administration), 72
Outpatient services, 17, 18–19, 55, 56–57

P

Panels, 71, 94
Parasitic diseases, ICD-9-CM coding for, 23
Parentheses (ICD-9-CM), 12
Past medical history (PMH), 53
Pathology and Laboratory codes (CPT), 37,
    71–72, 79
    panels, 71, 94
    reporting, 72
    structure and modifiers, 71
Patient examinations, documentation of, 54
Perinatal period conditions, ICD-9-CM coding
    for, 29
PMH (past medical history), 53
Poisoning, ICD-9-CM coding for, 32
Pregnancy
    CPT Surgery coding for, 68
    ICD-9-CM coding for complications, 28
Preventive medicine services, CPT codes, 57
Primary diagnosis, 17, 20, 92–93
Primary procedures, 43
Private payers, coding compliance, 86
Procedure codes, 34–79. *See also* CPT codes
    introduction to, 36
    linkage between diagnosis codes and, 84,
        87–88, 92

Professional component (CPT), 46–47, 63, 69
Puerperium complications, ICD-9-CM coding
    for, 28
Punctuation
    CPT codes, 42
    ICD-9-CM codes, 12–13, 25

R

Radiology codes (CPT), 37, 69–71, 79
    contrast material, 70
    reporting, 70
    special reports, 70
    structure and modifiers, 70
    unlisted procedures, 70
Reference labs, 65, 72
Referrals, consultations versus, 51
Respiratory system
    CPT Surgery coding for, 66
    ICD-9-CM coding for diseases of, 27
Respondeat superior, 89
Review of systems (ROS), 52–53
ROS (review of systems), 52–53
Rule-out diagnosis, 22

S

Secondary procedures, 43
Section guidelines (CPT), 40–41
Semicolons (CPT), 42
Sense organ diseases, ICD-9-CM coding for, 26
Separate procedures (CPT), 63
SH (Social history), 53
Signs, ICD-9-CM coding for, 21–22
Skeletal system. *See* Musculoskeletal system
Skin diseases, ICD-9-CM coding for, 28
Social history (SH), 53
Special reports (CPT), Radiology codes, 70
Specificity, coding to highest level of (ICD-9-CM
    codes), 22–23
Subcategories
    CPT (E/M) codes, 51–52
    ICD-9-CM codes, 10
Subclassification (ICD-9-CM), 11
Subcutaneous tissue diseases, ICD-9-CM coding
    for, 28
Subterms (ICD-9-CM), 6
Supplementary terms (ICD-9-CM), 6–7, 9, 14–16
Surgery codes
    CPT, 37, 60–69, 79
        auditory system, 69
        cardiovascular system, 66
        diagnostic procedures, 67
        diaphragm, 67
        digestive system, 67
        endocrine system, 68

eye and ocular adnexa, 69
    female genital system, 68
    hemic system, 67
    integumentary system, 66
    lymphatic system, 67
    male genital system, 67
    maternity care and delivery, 68
    mediastinum, 67
    modifiers, 63–65, 70–71
    musculoskeletal system, 66
    nervous system, 68
    operating microscope, 69
    procedures exempt from -51 modifier, 69
    reporting, 63–65, 94
    respiratory system, 66
    separate procedures, 63
    structure of, 60–62
    surgical package, 62–63
    urinary system, 67
    ICD-9-CM, 22
    surgical package, 62–63
Surgical package, 62–63
Symbols
    CPT, 43
    ICD-9-CM, 11–12
Symptoms, ICD-9-CM coding for, 21–22

T

Tabular List. *See* ICD-9-CM codes, Tabular List
Technical component (CPT), 69
Total body surface area (TBSA), 30–31
Training and education, coding and
    regulatory, 90
Truncated coding, 88
Turnover (carryover) lines (ICD-9-CM), 7

U

Unbundling, 58, 62, 89, 94
Undiagnosed conditions, 93
Unlisted procedures (CPT), 40–41, 70
Unspecified codes, 13, 88, 93
Upcoding, 88
Updating codes, 4, 5, 36–37, 90
Urinary system
    CPT Surgery coding for, 67
    ICD-9-CM coding for diseases of, 27

V

Vaccinations, CPT (E/M) codes, 73
V codes (ICD-9-CM), 14–15, 93

W

World Health Organization (WHO), 4, 13